THE POWER WITHIN

Record-breaking, ultrarunning and fighting for change

SOPHIE POWER

BLOOMSBURY SPORT

LONDON · OXFORD · NEW YORK · NEW DELHI · SYDNEY

BLOOMSBURY SPORT
Bloomsbury Publishing Plc
50 Bedford Square, London, WC1B 3DP, UK
Bloomsbury Publishing Ireland Limited
29 Earlsfort Terrace, Dublin 2, D02 AY28, Ireland

BLOOMSBURY, BLOOMSBURY SPORT and the
Diana logo are trademarks of Bloomsbury Publishing Plc

First published in Great Britain 2026

Bloomsbury Publishing Plc does not have any control over, or responsibility for, any third-party
websites referred to or in this book. All internet addresses given in this book were correct at the
time of going to press. The author and publisher regret any inconvenience caused if addresses
have changed or sites have ceased to exist, but can accept no responsibility for any such changes

A catalogue record for this book is available from the British Library

Library of Congress Cataloguing-in-Publication data has been applied for

ISBN: HB: 978-1-3994-2882-8; ePUB: 978-1-3994-2884-2; ePDF: 978-1-3994-2883-5

2 4 6 8 10 9 7 5 3 1

Typeset by Lumina Datamatics Ltd
Printed and bound in Great Britain by Clays Ltd, Elcograf S.p.A.

MIX
Paper | Supporting
responsible forestry
FSC® C018072

Bloomsbury Publishing Plc makes every effort to ensure that the papers used in the
manufacture of our books are natural, recyclable products made from wood grown
in well-managed forests. Our manufacturing processes conform to the environmental
regulations of the country of origin.

To find out more about our authors and books visit www.bloomsbury.com
and sign up for our newsletters

For product safety related questions contact productsafety@bloomsbury.com

For Donnacha, Cormac and Saoirse

CONTENTS

THE PHOTOGRAPH

My breasts are rock hard. I'm sitting on an uncomfortable plastic chair at the side of a crowded sports hall in Courmayeur, high in the Italian Alps. I set off from Chamonix, in France, at 6 p.m. last night. It is now 10 a.m. and I have been running for 16 hours. I'm exhausted. Around me are other runners, passed out on benches, getting some much-needed rest. Others are trying to eat, drink, tend to their feet or massage their tired legs. Most are surrounded by families and friends, rifling through overflowing sports bags looking for spare batteries, fresh clothing and food.

I need to do all this, but I have another job to do as well. My baby Cormac needs feeding and I have to express some of the milk that has built up since last night, causing me considerable pain. I sit quietly with him at the side of the room, as far away from the hustle as I can. It has been the longest time we've spent apart in the three months since he was born and I have missed him so much. My husband John tries to feed me an avocado sandwich while my friend Matt Hearne changes the batteries in my head torch ready for another night out on the mountain. Outside, my three-year-old son Donnacha is playing with our nanny Margita, waiting for me to come out and give him a hug before I head back on to the trail once more.

I'm trying to block out the noise of hundreds of people talking and hunting through bags of kit, which is reverberating loudly around the packed hall. Among the chaos of hundreds of bodies, I try to share a quiet moment with Cormac. I'm enjoying the change of priority away from putting one foot in front of the other up and down the mountains, my gaze not continually moving, looking for route markers to show me the way or hazards on the trail waiting to trip me up. For now, it is just me and my beautiful baby, connected to each other. Only three months ago he was living inside me. Now he's along for the ride as I take on one of the biggest ultramarathons in the world.

He is feeding quickly, as usual, relieving my painfully engorged breasts, which have been wondering where he was. Unfortunately, breastmilk production doesn't have a temporary shut-off switch. While I have been running my milk supply has kept apace, causing the skin to stretch tightly across my breasts.

At first it was tricky for Cormac to latch on. My nipples didn't have their usual softness and the buzz of noise around us is a distraction. But he is famished and I'm worried about contracting mastitis (inflammation of the breast tissue that can become infected), which is more likely if I don't feed regularly, so we work together in this crazy moment to relieve one another.

I express the milk from my other breast at the same time, so John can give him a bottle feed later. I need to multitask. I have limited time in which to complete the course and must soon head back out on to the mountain trail. I see a man speaking to John with a camera in his hand. Would I mind if he took my picture? He tells me he is working for Strava, a fitness app, telling the story of the race. He remarks that an athlete breastfeeding a small baby is an unusual sight. None of the other runners have even noticed what I am doing. Their field of vision is narrow and they are caught up in their own races, and their own priorities and problems.

John and I hesitate. This is a personal moment. But we know that these past months have been a struggle for me. We don't want other mothers to go through what I have had to in order to follow their dreams. Maybe this photographer can help change that. Running the Ultra Trail du Mont Blanc (UTMB), a 171km race around Mont Blanc, where you climb to over 10,000m, has been a dream of mine for many years. It's so popular in the ultrarunning community that to get a place in the race you have to accumulate points by running other ultramarathons and then be lucky in the lottery for would-be entrants. There are only 2300 places each year, limited by the capacity of the narrow, single-track paths and the impact of the runners on the fragile environment. I managed to get a place for the first time in 2014, but then became pregnant with my older son Donnacha. The race organisers refused to defer it to the year after, despite deferring places for injured runners.

Unlike injury, being pregnant, the race organiser said in a later interview, was a 'choice'. I was outraged, but powerless to object. It had taken almost a year to become pregnant with Donnacha and the timing was definitely not my choice. Unlike injury, pregnancy only happens to female runners, so it appeared to be seen as a 'self-inflicted medical condition'. Women already represent less than 10 per cent of entrants and this felt like another barrier to our participation; another way of saying we were of lesser value as athletes than the men we race alongside.

It took four more years until I was finally awarded another place. With two consecutive failed lottery entries for the UTMB, I was automatically guaranteed one the year after. I was already trying to get pregnant again, but my positive mindset assured me it would happen quickly. I estimated I'd have a year to train for the race after giving birth.

However, nature didn't take note of our plan. When I finally saw those two blue lines on the pregnancy test, I realised our baby would be only three months old when the race started. History was repeating itself. Again, I was not permitted to defer the place, but this is my dream, I thought, and I'm not going to let my chance pass this time. Not if there's any way I can make it happen.

We assumed the photo of me breastfeeding my baby would be a small story. Ultrarunning was still a fairly niche sport, after all. I hoped the organisers might see it and reconsider their policies, so I gave the photographer the green light and thought nothing more of it.

I spend the next few weeks in a daze being bombarded by media around the world. The photo has gone viral. What started as a simple post on the accounts of *Runner's World* and Strava has become a global phenomenon. It is being shared tens of thousands of times on social media and suddenly my name is synonymous with 'that breastfeeding ultrarunner'. I realise something groundbreaking is happening. Kathrine Switzer's 1967 Boston Marathon photograph, where officials tried to drag her off the course, proved how a single image could change women's sport. If hers opened the marathon to women, perhaps mine could open ultras to mothers. So I decide it's time to get to grips with Instagram, and start sharing my story. The real story. The one where I'm not a professional athlete, where I'm a working mum throwing balls up in the air hoping to catch some. The one where I create a support network around me to help me achieve my goals. The one where I run for my mental wellbeing as well as my physical health. And where I know that chasing my own dreams makes me a better mother.

I receive hundreds of messages and they continue to come. Often, they are from women trying to get back to fitness after having a baby or wondering how I exercised in pregnancy. They also come from fathers wondering how to better support their partners and women who are thinking about having children, but are worried about how to keep a part of themselves. But, most often, they are stories about the impact that seeing my photograph and journey since has had on them. About the confidence it has given them to pursue their goals and how it has lessened their maternal guilt when they take time out for themselves.

These are all feelings I struggle with myself. To this day, my life is a constant juggling act, but I have managed to find a way through the chaos. I am learning to balance family life with life-affirming challenges and driving positive change for others. Through these pages I want to share with you the story of an insecure teenager who came second to last in the school mile. The girl who never had any sporting role models and was never aware of her own ability. I'm not a naturally talented runner. My parents were never interested in sports and I was never encouraged to run or do any form of sporting activity. I was never picked for the school teams. And yet somehow, running found me. It has changed my path entirely, taking me on a wild adventure from the unsporty, overweight kid in school to the mother-of-three running for Great Britain and breaking down barriers for other women. To me, running represents escape, freedom, performance, advocacy, community and so much more. Through running I have discovered an inner strength and been able to hone in on my incredible internal engine. Running has taught me that sport can be a conduit to improve all aspects of our lives. It has given me lifelong friends around the world and a sense of community I'd never felt before. But most of all running is joy. I never regret lacing up my shoes, heading out the door and losing myself to the sound of pounding feet and trees moving in the wind. And it's these simple things in life that I cling to when everything else is swimming chaotically around me.

But I won't lie – it has been tough, with many mistakes along the way. As a mother I've had to carve out pockets of time and slot my training into cracks around my children's activities. I can often be found late at night working while heat training in the sauna. But I wouldn't have it any other way. None of us should be missing out on what brings us joy, whether that's my children's sports matches, my husband's cycling or my own quest to run across a country.

Fourteen-year-old Sophie Field would never have believed that less than three decades later she would be the owner of three GB running vests. And yet somehow this is where I ended up. This book is an attempt to share the story of where I began and where I am going now – because my journey isn't over. It also unpicks how this transformation occurred and what I've learnt along the way.

There have been two significant sliding doors moments in my life. The most well-known is that photo, which created a wave of events that changed my career and set me on a path to advocacy, and gave me the time and space to focus on performance. It ultimately led to me running for my country and setting two world records, one for the fastest crossing of the length of Ireland on foot and the other for the greatest distance on a treadmill in 48 hours. What is not as well known is that my first sliding doors moment came nine years earlier, when I jumped from non-runner to ultra-runner by signing up to a desert race on a whim. This led to a series of extraordinary adventures around the world and so many ultramarathons I have completely lost count of them (they are all in the appendix on p. 248 – at least the ones I remember).

While the role of motherhood plays a huge part in my story – it catapulted me into the spotlight after all – it is not my entire story. This book is not a guide on how to fit training and races around parenting. It is not a business or advocacy book on how I set up sports equity charity SheRACES, although it does high-light the injustices, inequality and sexism that provoked me to set up the organisation.

Instead, these pages serve as a map of my physical and psychological journey - charting how I became an ultrarunner, world-record holder, and advocate for change. They encompass the struggles and juggles of my chaotic family life, but also delve into something deeper. At the age of 43 I am at the peak of my sporting career. It might seem relatively old for an athlete, but it's taken me this long to truly unleash my inner power.

My third 24-hour World Championships lie ahead of me (they will have occurred by the time of publication) and writing this book has given me the opportunity to reflect on how I got here. It's a journey that takes in many rookie errors, an alarmingly close shave with death, an array of the world's toughest races (includ-ing Comrades, Spartathlon, UTMB and the Spine) and my desire to set two world records. It gives candid insight into what it takes to complete these challenges, and how to get to the start line. I have always struggled with the concept that I am a runner, and it has taken years to recognise that I am good at this stuff (and I still struggle to call myself an 'elite runner'). But somehow through it all I have been able to complete some incredible feats by continually testing myself and pushing my limits. Some of my challenges have been downright crazy (48 hours on a treadmill in front of a live audience!) and some have been hugely personal. But with every step I have learnt something about myself, about my performance and about the power we *all* hold within.

1
NOT A RUNNER

I remember the exact moment I attached the label 'I am not a runner' to myself; a label that remained tightly glued to me, an integral part of my identity, for over a decade. I was 14 years old, and my class were being led to the far sports field, where a four-lane running track was roughly painted on the scorched grass. We giggled and laughed as usual on the way over, but our mood quickly changed when we were told the session would start with running a full mile: Five and a bit laps of the 300m track. My idea of hell. I was over 11 stone, just five feet tall – and I absolutely hated running. I felt everyone was staring at my chunky legs and squidgy waist spilling over my constricting PE briefs. My size was helpful for shot put, javelin or discus – any sport I could put my weight behind – but I was not built for running. I tried to hide my anguish as we lined up for the dreaded mile. Just the far side of the track looked an impossible distance to me. Five circuits were going to kill me. I felt sick just thinking about it.

Clustered at the front were the few sporty girls, stretching their arms and bouncing on their feet. They looked excited, eager to see how fast they could run. The rest of us stood in the sunshine, sweating with fear, wanting to get it over and done with. I prayed for the earth to swallow me up as the teacher shouted 'Go!' Instead, I was jostled forward by the wave of girls and quickly pushed my way to the inside lane to minimise the distance I had to run. Within minutes I fell behind, panting by the first back straight.

By the second lap my navy gym briefs had ridden up and my thighs were being scratched by the unforgiving material as they rubbed together. My stiff pale blue polo shirt started to itch at the neck, reacting to the sweat. I shuffled along uncomfortably, trying to run with a wide gait to keep my thighs apart. Now I was being lapped, first by one, then by others, but my legs just could not carry me any faster. By the last lap there was only one girl behind me, the only one heavier than me in the class. Finally, I limped over the finish line, collapsing into the shade, underneath one of the giant trees that circled the field. My friends were grouped together already, chatting away, but I couldn't face them yet. I was embarrassed and sore, nursing a red mark between my legs. I felt exposed. My physical weakness had never been more apparent.

That muggy June day on a Surrey playing field, my fate was decided. *That. Is. It. Forever. I am not a runner.* I metaphorically wrote it on a white sticky label with permanent marker and superglued it to my chest, hidden underneath that stiff polo shirt.

I'm not sure why I expected to be able to run more easily, given that I never had. I'd never really taken part in sport, bar the mandatory sessions at school, and I'd never seen my parents play anything either. They had no interest in sport and it wasn't a part of family life.

What my father did do, though, is never slow down for me when walking, so I developed a very fast walking speed from an early age (learning to walk fast is the top tip I give anyone embarking on their first ultramarathon). It was only once I finally started running that my mother mentioned my beloved grandmother was once a cross-country champion, and that she herself was a sprinter at school. I was the complete opposite, labelling myself unsporty long before that fateful mile. My weight had perhaps been a contributing factor.

I first became aware I was larger than average when I was about six years old. My mum was a talented, graceful ballerina in her youth and took me to lessons, despite the obvious differences in our bone structure. At one class we were trying on costumes for the show. The teacher sifted through the pile, but none of the outfits fitted me. Eventually they resorted to putting me into an older boy's costume.

Then at age nine I overheard my grandparents discussing my weight with my parents. My grandfather called me over. 'Now, Sophie. I have a deal for you. If you lose 10 pounds I will give you 10 pounds.' Absolutely mortified, I ran to my bedroom trying not to let them see me cry. His offer didn't incentivise me – it was the complete opposite. I ate even more to comfort myself.

By age 10 I was pulled out of swimming because I wasn't fit enough to manage the eight-length warm-up. But the humiliation of the school mile switched something on inside me. Over the next six months I lost significant weight by restricting my calories and excessively exercising each night in my bedroom on a mini trampoline. My parents both worked long hours, and I took myself to school by train each day so they didn't notice what was happening, only that I was losing some weight. It was only when a friend at school intervened that I started to eat more normally – luckily before it developed any further.

At this point exercise was simply a way to control my weight, balancing out my love of food. Knowing the calorific values of everything (this could be my Mastermind subject) became useful later in life when I used it to inform my ultra fuelling strategies. But learning them aged 14 meant that for decades I was imprisoned by a mathematical formula. Every time a number on the scale was higher than a random figure I'd decided was right, I felt deflated. Despite being a healthy weight, I continued to feel ashamed of my body. I also continued going to great lengths to avoid running.

As the years went by that mile developed into several, via school cross country – on a route of our choosing. I chose the route that went straight across the road to my friend's house, where we watched *Neighbours* on TV and stuffed ourselves with pizza for an hour. Slinking back to school, we huffed and puffed, feigning tiredness to avoid detection.

The strange thing was, during all this time I really enjoyed sport, with the exception of running. I was quite the football fan, supporting Wimbledon FC and naming my pet gerbils Vinnie and Jones. And despite my lack of ability on the track I had always loved the outdoors.

My grandmother lived in Seascale on the edge of the Lake District and we'd spend our holidays hiking, wild swimming and playing on the beach. It was a rugged world away from the comfortable sandy hills of Surrey. I learned campcraft and survival skills, as well as developing a sense of belonging in nature. We would go on long hikes with my border collie Bonnie trying to make sure she didn't round up the sheep. It was never exercise, just an adventure in the outdoors. My much older cousin was a Scout leader and taught me from an early age to read an Ordnance Survey map. For each of our hikes in the fells I would have to write a route card, with estimated timings, checkpoints and escape routes identified, as well as go through the emergency kit and fuel we needed (always including pies from the local bakery in Gosforth – and a Mars bar, although it will still take a real emergency for me to eat one). I loved being active and longed to play team sport, but the clubs were invite only, those invites only coming if you had potential to make the school team. So I threw myself into music, playing the trumpet where my team sport was that of orchestras, wind bands, jazz bands and the like.

Just as the fells had taught me resilience and independence, my family showed me that strength was also about service, and that giving your time mattered more than anything else. From a young age, I saw that helping others wasn't optional, it was simply what you did.

My dad may have been hard on me but he was always soft on others. He spent his spare time taking children with disabilities swimming with my brother and me in tow, showing me how much joy a small act could bring. As a small child I'd hop on the minibus to help take partially sighted people to activities, proudly sitting behind my volunteer dad.

Meanwhile, my mum threw herself into local fundraising and later into the charity Smart Works, helping women rebuild confidence to return to the workplace. She had a gift for making women feel they belonged. As members of the Round Table and Ladies Circle, my parents were always busy helping those in need, and I was there by their side filling food hampers, quietly observing. I absorbed it all without realising: the idea that our time and energy have most value when they're used for others.

When he was not busy volunteering, my father worked as a gliding instructor at the weekends, and the only time I really got to spend with him one-on-one was on the airfield. I learned to fly at the age of nine, going solo at 16, which was the earliest possible at the time.

Gliding solo was my escape from the world. I could sing with no one to hear (except the time I accidentally held the radio button down), and glide from thermal to thermal for hours on a summer's day. It was the same meditative feeling I would discover years later on the trails. As my weight continued to fall during my teens, I gradually built confidence and decided to join 11F Air Cadets, and this youth arm of the Royal Air Force rapidly became my sanctuary.

Twice a week I would don my freshly pressed uniform with mirror-shined shoes and take part in a range of activities: anything from learning, and then teaching, the principles of flight to leadership, team building and outdoor survival. I found friendships hard to navigate at school as I never wanted to be in just one group of girls, toeing the party line, but in the cadets I could truly be myself. By sixth form I had risen to become Head of the Squadron, winning the county's Cadet of the Year award, partly for my work on inclusion, supporting cadets from less privileged backgrounds to pass their exams.

My love for exploration and the outdoors continued to flourish, and by the time school ended I was off on a hiking adventure before university. With no money to go on holiday abroad with the rest of my friends, I decided to do Wainwright's famous coast to coast hike with my cousin. The 306km trek from St Bees to Robin Hood's Bay is usually done in 18 days – but we decided 11 would be challenging yet doable. I was barely active, bar hauling tyres around at the gliding club, but in my mind it was just a

long hike. I never considered the idea of training for it or entertaining the fact I might not be able to physically complete it. We
rough-camped most nights, carrying large heavy packs due to
a lack of resupply points as we hiked over the Lakes, Dales and
Moors. On the third day I fell in a stream and could barely climb
out, so laden was I by my sodden pack, but the sense of achievement at the end was real and pure – and fish and chips had never
tasted better. It's amusing recalling this now, as today I could run
it in a little over two days (albeit without a 20kg pack).

Suddenly the summer was over and it was off to the University
of Oxford. I had secured my place reading philosophy, politics
and economics (PPE) at Christ Church, one of the most well-
known colleges. Back then it was known for its connections with
Alice in Wonderland author Lewis Carroll and 11 prime ministers.
Now it is far more famous as a location for the Harry Potter
films. I had applied mostly based on prettiness and cost of lodg-
ing rather than realising its heritage, and when my first tutorial
partner turned up in a tweed jacket and bow tie I wondered if I
had applied to the right place. While still moving in, my neigh-
bour enquired as to which school I'd come from, and as it wasn't
sufficiently prestigious she proceeded to ignore me for the rest
of our time there. Fortunately, my friend, (and future godmother
to my son) Rona, in the room on the other side, had suffered
the same fate and we bonded over our lack of upper-class-ness.

Thankfully the college is no longer as stuck up as it used to
be. During my time there the walls were adorned with the oil
paintings of men, representing an educational space that, shock-
ingly, was closed to women until as late as 1980. These days it is
far more inclusive and has made a conscious effort to encourage more female applicants.

A few years ago, the college commissioned several photographic portraits of high-profile women alumnae and I was
honoured to be one of them. There I stand in my Team GB
kit front and centre of Porter's Lodge. The first thing anyone
sees when they come into the college is a female symbol of
strength and sport. I'm glad to see that things have moved

forward; during my time there, I never felt I quite fitted into this strange environment and instead found my world outside, in the University Air Squadron (as I did with Air Cadets outside school). I woke up early to fly before lectures once or twice a week as I went through pilot then navigator training, with the goal of joining the RAF once I graduated.

Back on the ground I found myself dragged into college sport. The women's rugby and football teams were always short of numbers, so luckily for me there was no real selection criteria. I was made to feel I was doing them a favour just for showing up and standing there. My naturally strong build made me good at tackling, which partly made up for my lack of ball-handling skills.

I also joined a rowing crew, though mostly for the opportunity of crew dates with men's boats from across the university. I found that as part of a team I could push myself hard and I thrived on accountability to others. However, the label 'not a runner' was still so deeply ingrained within me that I took active measures to avoid the mile run to the boathouse. I got up early and walked rather than running there with my rowing crew. Somehow that school mile had imprinted in my mind that I couldn't run further than the length of a rugby pitch – and a half-sized one at that. And yet I was quite happy to take on endurance challenges within the Air Squadron, including the four-day 160km march in Nijmegen in the Netherlands and the mid-winter Tough Guy event in a village in Staffordshire. This involved a huge obstacle course with underground tunnels filled with freezing water.

Despite all my activity, I was also still struggling with the notion that I was overweight (I was a size 8), and signed up for the university gym to control the arbitrary number on the scale. Still harbouring the trauma of the embarrassing school mile, I could never bring myself to use a treadmill, opting for the cross trainer and static bike instead. The gym was not there to make my body stronger, as it is now, it was just a place to control my weight in a world of daily three-course dinners with wine.

The label 'not a runner' felt impossible to rip off, and prevented me from going for a run or loving my body for the incredible feats it could accomplish. Without realising it, I was placing restrictions on my ability, confidence and future opportunities.

On leaving Oxford University I went straight to my first role in the City as an investment banker at Morgan Stanley, having interned there the summer before. I'd made the heavy-hearted decision not to join the Royal Air Force. My brother was in the army, frequently deployed on overseas operations, and my father strongly advised me not to do it. Since it was the first time he had actually intervened in my life I decided I should probably listen.

Instead, I joined the dizzying world of mergers and acquisitions, working 100-hour weeks with weekends usually spent in the office. I had no control over my time. I longed to join a rugby team, but leaving the office at 11 p.m. most nights precluded it, so I resorted to infrequent sessions in the company gym at odd hours of the day.

I was regularly working all-nighters in the office, which would put me in good stead when it came to 100+ mile races in the future (and I'd much rather be running through the night in the mountains than pouring over an Excel model until dawn). As tough as it was, being an investment banker instilled a diligent work ethic in me to get the job done. It taught me life skills that I have taken out of the boardroom and on to the trails.

Two years later I went to study for an MBA (a Master of Business Administration) at the world's leading business school, the INSEAD (Institut Européen d'Administration des Affaires). I had an incredible year living in France and Singapore, working and playing hard, and exercise was barely on my radar. With English as my first language (unlike most of my peers), and a background in economics and finance, most of the harder classes came easily and, in my classmates' words, I 'partied on to the Dean's list.' I was in the top 10 per cent of my class, yet I seemed to spend more time having fun and 'networking' rather than studying. I still worked damn hard but I was already programmed to be efficient with my time. Without an exercise regime beyond opening champagne bottles with a sabre, I had no way to offset my love of French food (and wine) and put on a fair bit of weight.

It wasn't until my return to the UK that I started to think about my health again. I started work at a private equity company in Mayfair, where I often walked past a posh personal training gym. Passing it for the hundredth time, I had a lightbulb moment and decided to get myself a trainer. I was allocated Carl, a recently qualified trainer with a background in martial arts and weightlifting.

His sergeant-like nature was exactly what I needed. He soon realised I was strong for my size and had a particular talent for punching very hard. With a focus on my diet alongside the training, the weight quickly dropped off. I loved lifting and hitting the pads so hard the sound reverberated throughout the gym. Finally, I had found something physical where I could excel. Training became a regular part of my routine and, for a brief while, I somehow managed to find the time to work out once a week.

I found myself, age 24, excelling at work and life. My Mayfair job was in the retail space which I felt a strong affinity to. The firm's goal was to purchase chains of stores and make them more profitable before selling them for more. I threw myself into the role. I had worked in stores since I was 15 and became the link between the often out-of-touch financiers and those in the retail companies we bought.

At 25 I was named the *Harper's Bazaar* and *The Times* Young Businesswoman of the Year for making my name in a man's world. I told *The Times* newspaper that attitudes towards women in investment banking were changing thanks to senior women being less likely to tolerate discrimination. And I observed how women and men negotiated differently, with men more likely to storm out of a room if they were unhappy with their bonus.

My private life was flying too. Back when I was an intern I'd met John Power and we'd had a brief fling. Once we were both in full-time work we rekindled our relationship, moving in together within months. John was working in finance, too, and living together was the only way we could catch a glimpse of each other a few times a week. We worked in the same company, in buildings connected by a bridge, yet we never saw each other until late at night. We shared a work canteen but there was no chance we would ever sit and eat lunch together. Instead, each afternoon we both individually grabbed some food and ate at our desks. In the evening it was the norm to order takeaway and continue working. As mad as it sounds, the only possible way we could see each other was if we moved in together. John was a talented sportsman, having played tennis to a high standard in his youth, but frequent exercise fell away for him as well. We were both lost in the world of work.

When we did manage to have a few days off, we travelled to the Lake District to visit my grandmother and explore the fells. Our first overseas holiday took us to Morocco, where we climbed Mount Toubkal. The mountains were our shared love, with every hike drawing us closer together. So when it came to proposing to me, John knew a summit was the right location. Cleverly he chose Kilimanjaro in Tanzania, where I didn't have much time to think about my answer. Seconds after he bent down on one knee he was holding my hair back as I vomited everywhere. High altitude clearly didn't agree with me.

Our honeymoon in Brazil was another great escapade. We hiked in Chapada Diamantina, rode horses on reserves and snorkelled with dolphins. We shared our sense of adventure and longing for the outdoors. Everything was perfect. We were high flying in our finance careers and adventuring in the precious few weeks we had outside them. I was physically strong and enjoying my gym sessions. I felt on top of the world. But just when I least expected it, life turned around and bit me.

A few months after getting married, the situation at my firm changed. Our backers wanted us to reduce costs and I was selected as the one to be made redundant. It soon became clear that all the accolades and all my work could not make up for a ring on my finger. There was a choice between two of us: the other associate had a wife and kids to support, whereas I'd just got married and John had a good job. The implication was that I had John to support me so I didn't need the money, unlike my colleague. At the redundancy meeting I was told by a director that because I was now married, I should take the time to have babies (I was 26). And, of course, after that my brain would 'turn to mush' for a few years, so I should take an extended break from work. Up until that point he had been a supportive mentor, teaching me and pushing me to the top of my game, but he genuinely believed that, as a woman, I would be happiest having children and being a stay-at-home mother like his wife.

The whole situation plunged me into an existential crisis and things started to spiral downhill fast. My whole identity, confidence and sense of self was tied up with my career, which in one fell swoop was ripped out from under me. I was angry and frustrated about what had happened, and what that meant for my future. I didn't come from a wealthy family, I had earned my place and naively thought my sex was irrelevant; but all my assumptions – that in the workplace I was viewed as an equal, that being a woman didn't have to hold me back, that the world had moved on and there were no barriers to achieving my dreams – had been blown out of the water and my belief system was in tatters. I wasn't ready to become a mother – and certainly not to give up the career I'd worked so hard for. I didn't even know if I wanted children or not. I was no less capable for having changed my name from Field to Power. If anything, becoming a 'Power' should have been a win, so why was it being held against me?

I needed to escape and rebuild my shattered confidence. I turned to the only other thing I knew – exercise. At the first session after my redundancy meeting, Carl took out the pads and let me hit them until I cried. The action was incredibly cathartic and I knew I was on to something.

One of the amazing things about studying at INSEAD was that I developed friendships all around the world. At our wedding two of my three bridesmaids were classmates – from Ecuador and Costa Rica – and people flew in from all over the world to celebrate with us. A few weeks after I had been made redundant, John and I were due to head to Delhi for my friend Vaibhav's wedding. In a moment of madness while packing I cancelled my return flight, packed my 16oz pink boxing gloves and booked an onward flight to Phuket. I was going to punch and kick out my anger in a Muay Thai camp – and specifically learn to kick as high as the head of the firm (luckily he was only about five foot four).

John told me to come back when I was ready. He knew the toll the redundancy had taken on me mentally and that Thailand (and punching things) was as good as any place to sort my head out. One of my regrets had been not taking a gap year. My father – probably rightly – worried I would leave on an adventure, get distracted and never finish my studies, but this was a chance for a real change of scenery and to distract myself from the events of the past month.

Life at camp was pure and simple. I'd wake up at 6.30 a.m. and have a quick breakfast before two hours of group training followed by an hour of stretching. At 10 a.m. I had an hour of one-to-one coaching before an early lunch at a local restaurant. From 1 p.m. to 3 p.m. we had free time to cycle to the beach or take a nap. Then we were back to group training at 4 p.m. before a Thai massage at 6 p.m., a chicken cashew stir fry and bed. Monday to Friday were always the same, with one beach training session on a Saturday morning and Sunday off. All I had time to do was eat, train, recover and sleep. It was the perfect prescription for the state I was in.

The camp was mostly filled with Westerners but some locals trained there as well, meaning I had a mix of sparring partners. Saturday nights were fight night in Phuket Town and we'd all jump into the truck to drive down to watch. I hadn't ever planned on fighting, but my boxing background and strength gave me an edge over the local Thai girls who preferred to trade kicks – that and being a southpaw (left-hander), which they weren't used to fighting. I acted as sparring partner for several fighters at the gym and after six weeks of training I was readying myself to fight.

But it wasn't to be. I called John to tell him of my plans, and he gently suggested I might be ready to come home and find a job. I think he knew I'd struggle to hurt anyone physically and we'd long ago booked a hiking holiday in the Lake District for

Easter that he was looking forward to. Eight weeks after leaving Delhi, I returned home in the shape of my life.

Back in London I was still wondering what to do with myself. I was living off my redundancy pay and needed to figure out what to do next. Muay Thai continued to be my saving grace. Escaping to Thailand and developing a newfound physical confidence had helped to rebuild the self-esteem my redundancy had shattered. I might be seen as nothing more than a wife, but I was perfectly capable of kicking my former boss in the head.

I joined the local Muay Thai gym and met Danielle, who was a similar standard to spar with. She was retraining as a nutritionist, so we were both at a crossroads in life, and with the long walk to the gym (despite being incredibly fit, I of course never tried to run it!) our training occupied a lot of my days.

But being back in London with the pressure of finding a job was taking its toll. I shied away from social circles where the first question was always 'what do you do?' I took some advice from the wonderful Heather McGregor (otherwise known as the *Financial Times* writer Mrs Moneypenny), who had given me the business-woman award just a couple of years earlier, and decided to study for my accountancy exams.

This started to give structure to my days, but I needed more control over my destiny. The job search was frustrating – there was little out there that interested me and I was losing confidence in my ability to succeed in anything. I needed a challenge I could work towards: where I was the one holding the power, where aspects I could not control – like being a woman – were not barriers to success, and where I could prove my inner strength to myself and begin to see myself in a new light.

Coda: Not a runner

Throughout my young life, I placed countless labels upon myself without even realising the weight they carried. I believed I was 'fat' and 'not a runner' long before I'd even given myself a chance. I'd internalised these ideas so deeply that they shaped every decision I made – what I ate, what activities I tried, what I dared to imagine for myself. I thought real runners were thin, fast and looked nothing like me, so I stayed in my lane, convinced there were things people like me simply couldn't do. It took years to unpick those assumptions; years to realise that being a runner isn't about size, or speed or fitting a mould. Letting go of those labels was the key to a life I never thought I could have. I just had to open the door.

2
SAY YES

Marathon des Sables, Morocco

One Sunday in April 2009 I was watching the London Marathon. I had a rather sore head from the night before and was waiting on John to get out of the shower so we could make the 11 a.m. cut-off time for ordering bacon sandwiches at our local café. I remember wondering how they could possibly run for that long – three, four, five and more hours. I had been forced by the head Muay Thai trainers to attempt the short run to beach training in Thailand every Saturday, but had always given up after a few minutes and jumped in the wagon that followed the runners to the beach. I was still training with my strength trainer Carl, but avoided all pressure to use the treadmill, warming up instead on the cross trainer. I wasn't a runner, but I could kick someone in the head and that was enough for me. And yet bizarrely, somehow, three months later I'd signed up to run 250km across the Sahara Desert with just nine months to prepare.

Saying yes to this crazy adventure turned out to be another sliding doors moment as monumental as agreeing to *that* photograph being taken at UTMB; and it had all come about over a summer catch-up with a friend. While thousands of people were preparing to run 26.2 miles across the streets of London, one of my University Air Squadron classmates had been racing in the Marathon des Sables. I'd sponsored him, and as he was in

London that July, he wanted to take me to lunch to say thank you. Simon (or Harry as we called him due to his surname being Ramsden, like the fish and chip shop) was over a foot taller than me with an accompanying long stride. This had caused us both some problems when we marched together at Nijmegen, covering over 40km a day for four days in tortuous army boots (although some crazy Dutch people do it in clogs). Marching in step meant I had to stride out as far as I could, while he took tiny, awkward steps. Despite this barrier, we'd both loved the camaraderie of the event, the endless singing of songs that got ruder as each day went on, and the evening beers with military contingents from across the world.

As we chatted over lunch, Simon told me how he had walked most of the Marathon des Sables. He thought I was just as good a hiker as he was and would need no more endurance than I had for Nijmegen, so he reckoned I could easily finish the course. He told tales of the beauty of the desert and being alone under the stars during the longest stage. At the centre of his story were the strong bonds he built with tent mates and he convinced me that despite the pain in his feet it was one of the greatest experiences of his life.

In one of those 'screw it' moments I left the lunch and immediately called a charity that still had places for the next race. This was the opportunity I'd been looking for to take control and prove to myself that I was strong and capable. Without fully understanding what I was signing up for, I committed to raising £5000 and secured my entry. At this point I hadn't looked at what the race entailed. I hadn't even spoken to John. Something was telling me this was the challenge I needed to get me out of the hole I was in. I knew I needed to say yes.

The Marathon des Sables has been called the toughest race on earth (it's far from that, but it's an effective marketing slogan for its target audience). It is a race of 250km, over six stages – one of which is over 70km – through the Sahara Desert in Morocco. Temperatures range from below freezing to almost 50 degrees Celsius. As if that isn't difficult enough, competitors are forced to carry everything they need for six days, except for water and a basic canvas shelter. The list is daunting: food and a means to cook it, clothing, sleeping bag, mat, first aid kit, foot kit and the most useless waste of £5 I've ever spent – a venom pump. The cost of the race alone is around £2700 today, and that's before you factor in flights, food and specialist equipment. Once I'd paid my (large) deposit, the reality of what I had committed to hit me. While I knew that the emphasis on lightweight gear and good self-discipline played to my strengths, hiking for hours in the blistering heat was not going to be fun. I needed to save time and learn to run.

At this point I was living in Shoreditch in east London, which didn't have easy access to open trails. I had to weave through the crowds on Brick Lane, cut through Bethnal Green, and finally hit Victoria Park and the canal, which then went on for miles. And I knew absolutely nothing about running. Only that I had to. In vain I googled training plans and race plans, but found little that seemed designed to help me cope with the event's particular challenges, so I just laced my (shiny new) trainers up and went for a jog.

That first shuffle, T-minus nine months, was 10km, with a bit of walking in it. My legs weren't used to it, but thanks to the Muay Thai I was aerobically fit. It had also thankfully helped strengthen my weak right ankle, which I had broken badly at university playing rugby. A high tackle had sent me crashing down while my studs stayed rooted in the ground, twisting my foot violently. Since then, my ankle had been prone to swelling, but Muay Thai had unwittingly rehabilitated it. The pivoting and spinning on my grounded right foot (a core part of the discipline) built up stabilising muscles, ultimately saving my running career before it had even started.

As I started running more, and began a long commute to my new role, my Muay Thai training dwindled. I was running Financial Planning and Analysis for TK Maxx Europe, the discount store brand, and enjoying working in retail. There were no super-rich egos to contend with, like I was used to in finance, and I didn't have the daily struggle of questioning the values of what I was doing. I was back to working for the customer as part of a team of genuinely decent staff members, but the thing that had saved me – Muay Thai – was now slipping away. I had fallen out of love with sparring against six-foot-plus men who couldn't control their strength. Luckily, my training partner Danielle was also a runner and helped me through those first painful miles. I eventually joined a gym and started running on a treadmill for two minutes fast with a walking rest for a minute, repeating 10 times. I'd seen a workout like that on a *Runners' World* training plan, and it felt challenging enough.

Two months into training I entered the Run to the Beat Half Marathon in London, which some of John's friends were doing. John had decided to sign up too as he had just started training for triathlons – so I opted to join them. For John and his mates, it was an excuse to run in the morning and then sit in the pub all afternoon. I wanted to come along for the ride. I had no idea what to expect, but I had covered the distance in training, so I knew I could finish – I just had no pacing strategy.

Despite my significantly greater run training volume, John decided he was going to sit on my shoulder for the entire race. And sit. And sit. This got really annoying after a while. I felt like his personal pacer rather than someone running their own race. I knew I should be faster given all my training and finally understood that, if he was still with me, I had gone out too slow. I accelerated away leaving John behind as he blew up on a hill and started to walk. I finished in 1:49:01 (John limped in at 2:01:05), and I realised that was a pretty good start to my running career. I had naturally paced well through the crowded streets despite being clueless as to what I was doing. I had no real strategy and didn't fuel during the race – I simply ran. Crossing the finish line I was absolutely buzzing and headed straight to the pub to celebrate. Maybe running wasn't so bad after all. But I also knew the Marathon des Sables was an entirely different beast. It wouldn't be about speed – it would be about survival.

Next, bypassing the full marathon distance, I signed up for my first ultra, the Druid's Challenge run by XNRG, a well-trodden training ground for would-be Marathon des Sables entrants. The event follows a long-distance path of 136km from Tring in Hertfordshire, along the Chilterns, to Avebury in Wiltshire. The race was spread over three days, with nightly accommodation in school sports halls. It was my first test of whether I could run, not just hike, over multiple days and I hoped to meet other runners who were also headed to Morocco and see what I could learn from them.

I realised I'd need some trail shoes, so I went to a running store a few days before the race – a massive rookie error – and packed them straight into my bag. Ten miles into the race something hurt on the back of my heel. I took my shoes off and discovered they were covered with blood. I still had 122km to go.

Luckily, I encountered an RAF medic volunteer who cleaned and dressed both my heels every night. My feet became quite the tourist attraction as we all got ready to sleep, because the cuts developed into large flesh wounds, and I had to run-limp through the remaining days. It was a silly mistake, but I thought of the pain as good training for potentially worse disasters during the desert race. I discovered it helped when I let out a little squeal every time I started moving again, just until my feet were warmer and the sharp pain dulled a little. It helped knowing this wasn't my first rodeo with painful extremities. I'd had to kick-box in Thailand with cuts on my feet and endure blisters while marching for four days in Nijmegen. I was a pro at managing pain, but the new footwear mishap was a clear message that I had no idea what I was doing.

So I decided it was time to see Mr Marathon des Sables himself, Rory Coleman. Rory had run the race several times and had developed a coaching business getting novice runners like me round the course. His one-day training session involved running a slow marathon together while he doled out all the advice you needed. At the time there was very little information anywhere – no Facebook groups or WhatsApp communities – so

I needed all the help I could get. Rory's insights proved invaluable for many reasons – especially the 'sprint to the best tent' advice, where securing a tent close to the finish could save a lot of post-finish line pain.

However, I was taken aback when he told me to lose weight if I wanted to finish. I was a healthy size 8-10, and thought I had finally gotten over my weight demons. Being told I needed to be lighter was a knock to my confidence. Looking back now I feel it was a misguided thing to say to a young woman, no matter how honourable his intentions. It also didn't reflect the reality of the race when I got there, where many (mostly men) were carrying a few extra pounds and still managed to make it through to the end. While I did heed his advice and lost a few pounds, I also lost some of the body confidence I had taken so long to develop. Since starting to run I'd managed to free myself of the mental load of counting calories, of the continual feeling that my body was too big, but Rory's comments made me feel uncomfortable with my body shape once more.

My next ultramarathon (recommended by Rory as it was his own race) was utterly grim, although at least I'd found shoes that didn't try to strip flesh from my feet. Over two days and with one overnight stay (at least in a hotel this time), it covered 76km each day along a miserable canal. This was not a quintessential English towpath flanked by wildflowers and mild-mannered cows chewing the cud at the water's edge. It was a dank stretch along the murky grey Grand Union Canal from Northampton, and I spent the time counting shopping trolleys in the canal and trying not to get tripped up by fly fishers. It was a horrible weekend, but with two long back-to-back days I'd got a good amount of training in, and had my first experience of running in the dark with a head torch. With just four months to go until the big race this was all great preparation.

Running with a head torch was something I found strangely disorientating. I was using one of my old camping headlights, which had a narrow beam, and every time I turned to speak to the runner next to me I lost sight of the ground in front. This also led to missing a key turnoff on the first night, which only added to my misery. Since then, I've become used to running with a head torch and strangely it is also when I feel safest on the trails. No one can tell I'm a lone woman as my size and shape are obscured. To any onlooker I'm just a spotlight, running along the trails, and surely a woman wouldn't be out alone, so it has to be a man.

Another joy is being able to have an easy wild toilet stop. You just go a few metres off the path, turn off your torch for total privacy and do your business. This is much simpler than endlessly searching for a bush that may shield you, but which invariably pricks your bottom.

I had one final race planned before Marathon des Sables as a final kit test – the Pilgrim Challenge on the North Downs Way (along which I now live). This is a wonderful introductory ultramarathon race – 53 hilly trail kilometres from Farnham eastbound on the Saturday, staying overnight in a school sports hall and running back the next day. By this point I'd realised the value of packing a luxurious electric blow-up bed in my drop bag for the evening (as well as two eye masks and earplugs), so was rather looking forward to feeling smug later that day.

Unfortunately, the smugness never came. It had been raining heavily in the days before the race, and at 26km I skidded in the mud on a downhill stretch and immediately realised something wasn't right. I couldn't push off on my right leg and was limping badly. A runner behind me stopped and generously gave me one of his poles. Hobbling forwards I managed to make it to the next aid station a few kilometres away.

Luckily for me, my brother Adam wasn't too far away and for the promise of a free burger and chips he picked me up from the aid station. I knew I could have made it until the end of the day, but what would I have gained? I'd already proven my ability to go further than this race, and across three days, not two. This race wasn't my A race – the race that I really wanted to do well at. That was the Marathon des Sables itself, which was only six weeks away. With that as my focus, the sensible thing to do was not to cause myself any further damage. I had the fitness; I had the strength, I just needed to recover from the injury – which turned out to be a damaged hip flexor. Covering more kilometres that day would have taken me further away from my goal, rather than towards it.

I'm a firm believer in finding the silver lining to any setback. The bright shiny one from my Pilgrims injury was in three parts. First, I'd have more time to focus on the right kit. Second, I wouldn't be able to overtrain and if I let my hip heal properly would be going in fresh. And third, while in recovery I'd be doing more training appropriate to the Marathon des Sables, like walking on a treadmill up an incline.

Having the right kit in an ultra can sometimes be the difference between making it to the finish line or not. In stage races like Marathon des Sables, it takes on a much higher importance, because apart from water and basic shelter, everything you need for the seven days has to be carried in your rucksack. Take too little food or gear and you end up hungry and cold. Take too much and you are slowed down, resulting in extra hours exposed to temperatures of 40 degrees Celsius.

I have always been one for a good Excel spreadsheet and an optimised plan – Excel models were a big part of my work in mergers and acquisitions in my early days. As well as my background in trekking in the Lake District, learning military planning techniques has been very helpful in planning for ultras. I knew every gram had to count. My research opened up a whole fascinating world of weight-saving equipment designed for travelling light. I indulged in a customised sleeping bag – for exactly my height with the highest quality down. I even added extra warmth for my toes as I have Raynaud's disease, which means I struggle with keeping my hands and feet warm. I had to tell myself I'd use it many times on races in the future to justify the cost (I was at least right in this). My cutlery and cooking pot were lightweight titanium, and my stove came in at just 27g.

I even sawed off the end of my lightweight plastic toothbrush and took dried flakes of soap to wash with. My luxuries were minimal – a lightweight set of flip-flops for the camp (which I got free with a summer fashion magazine), an eye mask and ear plugs, and a teeny trial-size lavender sleep spray.

Food was the toughest to pack. The rules stated a minimum of 2000 calories per day (if I ran it again now I'd definitely take much more), but this meant the weight reached almost 3kg. I spent hours researching the calorific value per 100g of every foodstuff I would need throughout the entirety of the race. Gels – not that I liked them – were out due to their water content, which made them too low in calories per gram, as were simple carbohydrates. I learned that carbs and protein had four calories per gram, but fats had a whopping nine. That meant that the fattier the food, the more calories I could get for less weight. At the top of the pyramid were macadamia nuts at 800 calories per 100g, but I opted for cashews, because I preferred the taste, and they came in around the 700 mark. Freeze-dried 'dinners' averaged 500 calories per 100g and I found the chicken tikka option to be the most palatable. While running I planned to have chia flapjacks with a small bag of Skittles or wine gums for a sugar hit when I needed it. My evening treat was in the form of a little bag of Jelly Bellys or peanut M&Ms – the only chocolate that wouldn't melt and the nut centre pushed up the calorie density.

In the end my food averaged about 500 calories per 100g and I carried an average of 2200 calories per day. I'd be burning around 4000+ calories a day, so was looking forward to losing a good 3lb that I could enjoy putting on again at the end. I was so obsessed with the weight I was carrying that I even decanted all my freeze-dried food into lighter bags to save another 100g. Advice from Rory had been that I could saw off half of the water bottles I would be given by the crew with the small mandatory pen knife I had to carry. With this sawn water bottle, I could make a bowl to reconstitute the food each night rather than use the heavier foil packaging it came in. That wasn't the only sawing I would be doing. I attacked my backpack – cutting off all the strap length I didn't need. By the end of my DIY preparation, I had a pack weighing 7.5kg, excluding water.

During this prep time I was still unable to run while my hip flexor healed and I started to find hiking on the treadmill incredibly dull. My solution was to swap most of my gym time for hot yoga. The local studio had a '30 days for £30' offer, which I started 30 days before my flight to Morocco, and I was determined to get value for money. At my first session I felt horrendous and had to sit down during the class as the world spun around me, but gradually it started to feel much better. As a naturally nonflexible person who had neglected stretching since stopping Muay Thai (I could no longer kick my ex-boss in the head should the opportunity arise), it was difficult at first to discover I couldn't do most of the positions. Looking around I knew I was 'fitter' than most of those in the room – I could run further, faster, could lift more – so it felt frustrating to be 'bottom' of the class. But I kept telling myself the real purpose was to push myself to increase my heart rate in the heat and prepare myself for the conditions I would be facing.

Over the month I gradually became marginally more flexible, but, more importantly, I was able to tolerate the heat without feeling sick. Looking back, this is very similar to the way I prepared for the 24 Hour World Championships in Taiwan – this time advised by British Athletics sports physiologists rather than making it up!

Before I knew it, the time came to leave for Morocco. The British contingent in the 2010 race was one of the largest, alongside those from France, from where the race founder hails. There were so many of us that the Brits were accommodated on a separate charter flight to Ouarzazate. I saw a few familiar faces from the 'training' ultras and it was easy to pick the other runners out in the airport – everyone was dressed in running gear, and keeping everything they could for the race in their hand luggage to avoid losing it. I noticed that people were not only overwhelmingly male – around 90 per cent – but also an older crowd. I was 26, but the average age was probably two decades older and I felt a little uncomfortable. There was also a range of body shapes – certainly those who wouldn't look out of place on a marathon podium, but also those who didn't fit the 'norm' for an ultrarunner. The race has always been one to attract novice ultrarunners, especially since it is self-titled as one of the hardest races in the world, and many would argue it is often a mid-life crisis sign-up for desk-bound executives attracted by the challenge and bragging rights. On reflection, though, I'd also signed up mid-crisis – I'd just had mine much earlier in life.

When we arrived, the Brits were thrown together in a hotel in Ouarzazate and I was assigned to a room with a wonderfully cheery girl who was even smaller than me. She had run several marathons before, but this was also new territory to her. We spent that afternoon reassessing her pack and stripping it lighter. The more conversations I had, the more I realised that my kit prep at least had been a lot more detailed than others, with a much higher focus on minimising weight. That afternoon we had a quick briefing from the organisers on what would happen over the next few days. Once we returned to the hotel post-race, victorious or not, we were warned that the beautiful inviting swimming pool would be strictly off-limits to us. The reason given was that many of us would by then have infected feet. I shuddered. This was more detail than I wanted, but I made a mental note to look after mine as best I could.

We were told that tents during the race were allocated based on nationality, but you could choose who to share the eight-person tents with. I'd met a couple of the other competitors, James and Tom, at other training races, so we joined together. I asked them to find a few more friendly faces until we had our band of eight.

The next day we streamed into coaches and headed on a horrendous four-hour drive to the desert. The coaches were stuffy and there was an air of nervousness. From here on there were no drop bags (bags containing spare kit and nutrition to be accessed mid race) or shops for replacements. If you'd forgotten anything, that was that.

On a comfort stop the men lined up by one side of the coaches to pee while the few women all headed off road in search of a dried bush to crouch behind. Little did I know it, but this caution for our modesty would quickly disappear during the race. As the road ended we switched vehicles and climbed into a range of trucks headed over the rough terrain towards the largest circle of tents I had ever seen. On the advice of Rory I sprinted for a tent close to the entrance of the circle, number 108. The additional walk to the further tents might have been OK on day one of the race, but he had been clear that the early sprint would save a lot of extra pain come day three onwards.

They were the most basic tents I had ever seen – basically a large piece of cloth held up by poles with open ends. A carpet was laid on the sand, which we had to lift to remove stones from underneath. This helped to make things a little more comfortable given we were only on lightweight blow-up mattresses, most of which would eventually succumb to puncture from a stray thorn.

We had two nights in the tent before the race started, because it took that long to kit-check a thousand athletes. It was a good time to get to know the tent members I'd be going on the journey with, all with different stories and reasons for being there. It was the first Marathon des Sables for all of us, which I was grateful for as I wasn't sure I wanted to hear stories about what was to come. I was the only woman, and by far the youngest, but immediately felt comfortable being around them. The first night we were treated to a proper French dinner with wine and a cherry clafoutis for dessert, laid out on long tables. I found myself dreaming of that fruit days later, when the freshest thing I had were freeze dried strawberries in my gloopy porridge.

During the kit-check period we were handed roadbooks which described each stage. The total distance would be the longest ever for the Marathon des Sables – 250km for its 25th year over six stages. The route tended to change each year, but always followed the same broad format. The longest stage within it – stage four – was a double stage, where we would run almost two marathons back to back, with many of us expected to finish well into the second day. We did not have to map read – the course was very well marked – but the booklet described the stages, their terrain and when we could expect water stops. Water (and salt tablets), as well as a travelling tent, were the only things the organisers provided. The rest we carried ourselves.

I had no GPS watch – few runners did and I didn't cave and buy one until six years later – so I was relying on my £5 Casio to keep track of time and remind me when to eat. That night our tent members poured over the roadbooks, enjoying our last decent feed before we went on rations for the race ahead. A restless night's sleep followed as I tossed in the sand, excited and nervous in equal measure.

The morning start line was an incredible fanfare of loud music, jostling feet, and trying to listen to speeches in French and English. In the chaos I started chatting to a Costa Rican man who had asked me to take a picture. He'd decided to carry the extra weight of a camera, as camera phones weren't standard back then at all. I mentioned my Costa Rican friend Carolina, who had been a bridesmaid at my wedding, and a few details later we realised he'd been at school with her. I somehow felt a little less alone, and in the days to come I'd find other connections with runners from across the globe.

The first day was fairly short – just 35km. We set off, as we did every day, with AC/DC's 'Highway to Hell' blasting from the speakers. Hundreds of runners sprinted off the start line, forgetting the weight of their packs and the days ahead of them. I'd been advised by Rory to start at the back each day and work my way forward. This seemed a little too cautious, so I started in the middle, but every kilometre I began to pass people, which would be the same for the whole race. People picture the Sahara as miles of sand dunes – which sections of it are – but mainly it was runnable dried mud with a few rocks. I came home third in my tent, which would also remain the same for the rest of the race. In the first days, I never looked at where I was in the women's ranking, because it was entirely irrelevant to me. I only knew I felt good and was pleased that my meticulous preparation had paid off, especially all those hours of hot yoga, which meant I had somewhat acclimatised to the heat.

For many others, though, the first day was a wake-up call. The 35km that competitors could cover in training in three hours at home had taken well over five – in the heat, on the rocky sandy terrain and with a heavy pack. As my tent mates couldn't change the heat or the terrain, their packs were stripped down over the next two days. I was one of the happy beneficiaries of a lot of discarded food they realised they simply could not carry. This was a bit of a lifesaver as I hadn't realised that in a hot climate the last thing I'd be able to stomach in the morning was gloopy porridge. With the need for me to eat to keep my energy up, my tent mates had been resorting to feeding me spoon by spoon like a toddler with aeroplane sounds for effect. The excess food being removed from packs luckily allowed me to switch things up, as I found their jettisoned flapjack bars infinitely easier to keep down first thing – and with no need to boil water I could have more of a lie in.

While the days were long and hot, the race gave me a similar feeling to the simple life I had loved in Thailand. We had little food, barely any luxuries and were even limited on communications – we were allowed to send one email a day from the sweltering computer tents and receive one printout of messages from friends and family. Our focus was on running, eating and resting, with a bit of self-admin thrown in. I found it deeply moving how our tent came together as a team, despite having barely known each other before. Those of us getting in earlier took to helping the slower runners as soon as they arrived – heating their water for dinner, laying out their sleeping gear and helping with their feet.

Feet became our obsession. Blisters, cuts and infections are common and can prematurely end a race. Each morning, I would clip on the yellow parachute silk gaiters that came up to my knee and were glued around the edge of my trainers. Despite this, the sand still managed to get in, and most evenings I was tending to several new blisters – though I luckily escaped the worst of what I saw in my tent.

As the stages passed, I realised that I was gaining ground on others – I was told I had entered the women's top 20, despite taking every day cautiously and never pushing too hard. Finishing was the only goal, but I was efficient – quick at the checkpoints and I could out-hike some of the tallest men. As the heat rose to 47 degrees Celsius, I managed to keep a good hiking pace, becoming particularly strong during the long stage. I joined up with two guys, including a very funny American called Jimmy who shared my love of peanut M&Ms. We fast-hiked through the night, following light beams from point to point, and finished in just 15 hours, around midnight, giving us a full rest day.

It would be late the following afternoon that my tent mate Tom arrived after a second full day in the heat. Tom, who worked in electrical utilities building substations, was a recovering alcoholic who had started running to help him stop drinking. He had been dry for almost two years and this race signified, if not the end of his struggle, a strong marker that he was able to get there. Years later I scheduled a business trip to New York so I could run the penultimate leg of Tom's run across America with him. In non-ultra life, a City-working Oxford graduate was never likely to meet a recovering alcoholic from Yorkshire, never mind develop a close friendship, but I quickly found this to be the beauty of ultrarunning.

Every night we chatted as a tent – our mix including a primary school headmaster, psychologist, police officer, company director and consultant. It was a mix that was unlikely to come together in everyday life, but we shared something so deep and unforgettable via our race experience. Career, wealth or background was secondary – instead, competitors chatted about their shared love of running and conversations meandered down a myriad of unexpected passageways.

Through the pain and strain of running mile after mile, it was hard to maintain any sort of façade and we were all stripped back to our core essence. In the desert, where there was nothing to buy, money had no currency; the only currency was yourself and what you had in your pack. The simplest of gestures made a remarkable impact. When a runner was struggling to eat I offered him a pack of Skittles I'd plundered from a teammate lightening his pack a few days earlier. It gave him the boost he needed to be able to race again the next day.

I was also able to share my water with those that needed it most. We were restricted to two and half litres each and were issued with a water card to clock off our allocation. Every person received the same allocation – no matter their size. This actually gave the women, who tended to be smaller, an advantage over the men. At five foot three I didn't need as much water as Olympian rower James Cracknell (kipping in the tent next door), who literally towered over me.

While the men were struggling with the water rations, I had enough spare to wash some of my kit. At the end of each day, I squeezed my t-shirt and underwear into a zip-lock bag with water and soap flakes. It felt so good to have something clean for the next day. Any extra water I then left at the tent next door which was bursting with hulking guys. It was an example of how equality does not always translate to equity, so I wanted to do my small part to redress the balance.

I was also at the receiving end of kindness when I was struggling and in pain with a knee injury. While wandering around chatting to people in other tents each day post race, I'd made a strong connection with a girl called Ronnie. On the final day of racing she gave me one of her poles, as I had none, and stayed with me until the finish line. This small act enabled me to finish the race and she became one of my closest friends, despite living thousands of miles away in Dubai. Later, she moved to London and then we went through motherhood together, but I will never forget sharing a finish-line pizza with her in a tiny town in the middle of nowhere. It was the most delicious thing we had ever eaten.

I was the 19th woman to cross the line, 257th overall out of 1013 starters (and 923 finishers – proof it can't be the hardest race if over 90 per cent finish), and third in my W23 age category.

I marvelled at the women leading the race and celebrated that British woman Jen Salter (now Coleman) had made the podium. I would never have believed that 12 years later I'd be pulling on a GB vest alongside her. What I did know, however, was that the race hadn't been as difficult, mentally or physically, as I had imagined. There had been hard times, such as the never-ending long stage when we didn't quite know which light was the last route marker and would lead us to our beds. And then there was the hottest day, when even a shuffle run caused my body to overheat, forcing me to walk. But I never felt I was near any kind of personal limit. I'd prepared well, followed the process and just put one foot in front of the other efficiently. I felt I'd finally found a sport I was competent – if not good – at, but I still didn't see myself as a runner.

What stayed with me most from the Marathon de Sables was not the personal achievement, but the bonds I made. These types of event enable you to make the most amazing friendships. They break you down, which leads to true honesty between running companions and creates a safe space where thoughts can be openly shared. Running alongside complete strangers I chatted about the pros and cons of marriage, the difficulty of having kids and what to do about being bullied at work in a franker manner than I would with my closest friends, often after only knowing the person for a few hours. Many of these people I never met again, but each shared time on the trail with me that I treasure. The race was an experience like no other and set the stage for my life to come.

While for many of the runners finishing the 'hardest race on the planet' ticked a box, for me it opened a new door. If I hadn't simply said yes when Simon encouraged me to sign up for the race I may never have found running, but I had the gut feeling that doing something so alien, so scary and so overwhelming was the right thing to do.

When I landed back at Heathrow John met me carrying a big box of posh chocolates – far more useful to a runner in recovery than flowers – and he immediately knew something had changed. I had a new sense of confidence in myself and a belief in my own abilities to achieve the goals I set. I was ready to move forward.

Coda: Say yes

The Marathon des Sables was an experience like no other. From the scorching heat to the camaraderie of my tent mates, the race pushed me beyond anything I had known. I formed deep friendships, shared meals under the stars and found joy in the simplest of comforts – a handful of Skittles or a kind word of encouragement. The desert stripped away life's distractions, leaving only the raw essence of perseverance and human connection. By the time I crossed the finish line, tired but elated, I knew that saying yes to this challenge had changed my life. Running had become more than just a race – it was a journey, a discovery and a lifelong passion that had only just begun – and it had taught me that sometimes the best decisions are the ones that terrify us the most.

3
NEVER REGRET

Running into a coma, Cambodia

'Your wife has fallen into a coma. There's a 50 per cent chance she dies and a 50 per cent chance she survives with brain damage. You need to get on a plane right away.' No one should ever have to receive a call like this.

My husband John was 6000 miles away when the telephone rang. The emergency call was made by the lead medic on a 220km multi-day race I was competing in across Cambodia, which finished at the historic temples of Angkor Wat. I had severe hyponatremia, a condition where the levels of salt in the body are diluted. In an effort to avoid dehydration in the appalling humidity and heat, I had gone the other way and drunk too much water. This seemingly innocuous mistake had caused my brain to swell. I had collapsed in camp and was unconscious on a stretcher, awaiting a helicopter to take me out of the Cambodian jungle to hospital.

This was a holiday. I was 30 years old and meant to be having fun. And now it was 50-50 whether I even lived, with no chance given for a full recovery.

It had been a fairly last-minute decision to go to this Global Limits race in Cambodia in November 2012. By then I was fully immersed in the world of multi-stage races, the Marathon des Sables having ignited something deep within me. John and I had taken part in a trek across Nepal plus an incredible six-stage, 250km running race in Iceland – Fire and Ice. It was in Iceland that we met two other competitors, Canadians Simon Donato and Paul 'Turbo' Trebilcock, who were filming a series of adventure races around the world for a programme called *Boundless*. The other races in this series included mountain biking, paddle-boarding and triathlons, as well as a few ultramarathons – some single stage and some over multiple days, like in Iceland. Over the course of the race we became firm friends with them and their film crew, who followed us around the course, intrigued by how the stresses and strains of the race would affect our relationship.

The next race they were filming, a few months later, was to be in Cambodia and they suggested I join it. The format was the same as in Iceland – roughly 220km over six days, but this time we would only have to carry what we needed for the day, because our main kit would be transported between camps for us. In Iceland, as in Marathon des Sables, we had to carry everything we needed for the whole race, except our tent and water. Running with a heavy pack is physically demanding, but the greater challenge is often surviving with only the limited food and equipment you can carry. Having been constantly hungry (and therefore grumpy) in Iceland because I could not carry enough food for the colder conditions, the idea of a faster, happier (and warmer) race appealed. John had little interest – he had suffered in a hot triathlon the year before – but I had enough annual leave left and messaged the organiser straight away to book my place.

As soon as I landed in the capital city, Phnom Penh, the humidity hit me. John and I had been on holiday there a few years before, travelling across the country, discovering hidden temples and learning about their history – but I'd forgotten just how energy-sapping the water-logged air was. I thrived in the Marathon des Sables, in the dry Saharan heat, but this clamminess was a different case entirely; every breath felt laboured as if the oxygen was being sucked out of my body.

When I arrived at the hotel for the welcome dinner, I was excited to reunite with Turbo, Simon and the film crew – Josh Eady, his brother Jordan Eady and Steven Bray, the producer. I also started talking to a man named Krasse, a heavily tattooed chef from Bulgaria who had formerly been in the military. With his motivational catchphrases and no-nonsense approach he reminded me of an ex-boyfriend. I didn't know it then, but we would go on to become close friends and training buddies, with him crewing me out in Greece for the Spartathlon ultramarathon. He also put up with my endless pee stops during training when I was six months pregnant with Donnacha.

It had been a full 18 months since the Marathon des Sables, my last (and first) big solo adventure, and while I had loved racing with my husband in Iceland and Nepal I also longed to race alone again. Being by myself, without the security of John, made it easier to form new and deeper bonds with others. It was too easy for us to talk to each other when we had some down time – being alone forced me to reach out and chat to other people. I also felt it helped reconfirm my identity as just myself, outside of our partnership, giving me more confidence in my strength to stand alone. This point-to-point race was small, only 29 self-selected runners, 10 of whom were women from around the world, all with stories to share. While Turbo and Simon were clearly there to win, racing competitively each day, there was also a jovial group of Indian men along for the ride, whisky packed for party time each night. I was excited about getting to know everyone during the course of the race. In most single-stage events you only spend time with the runners around you, those who run at your speed, but in Cambodia we were going to have a full week together, with time in camp each night to truly connect with everyone. Faster runners would live alongside those who would be mostly walking the course.

Before our first day in camp we left the hotel for a tour of the city. Phnom Penh was an assault on the senses. There were people everywhere, and crossing the road reminded me of the old arcade game *Frogger* as we dashed, ducked and dived between bicycles, scooters and carts. Around every corner there was an exquisite temple with numerous towers constructed to mimic sacred mountain peaks. We stopped at a market where Simon dared me to eat a deep-fried spider's leg for the camera – something I would ordinarily never do, but being filmed it felt difficult to back down. Luckily it only tasted of the deep-fried coating and a quick gulp of water helped me forget it.

Later that day, following a four-hour bus ride to camp, I was interviewed about how I planned to push myself during the race and explore where my limits were. I have always pushed myself in some way during races, but it felt slightly different having a camera on me. I felt more pressure than normal, knowing that my performance would be documented and shown around the world, even if the focus of the film was on the Canadian duo.

Before setting off for the first stage we spent a night sleeping under individual pink mosquito nets, hung in rows inside a large farm building. Compared to the freezing tents of Iceland, being under cover here felt luxurious. The following morning we rose early and a group of local monks, a sight in their bright orange robes, sang to us and blessed our journey ahead.

By 8 a.m. the humidity was already immensely oppressive, but I was keen to keep moving efficiently. The first stage was a fairly gentle 30km to introduce us to Kampong Thom province. It couldn't have been more different to the desolation of Iceland. The red dirt road was awash with cows meandering free, while motorbikes and scooters weaved precariously between them. Simon and Turbo sped off at the front, alongside Salvador Calvo Redondo and Manuel Pastor, talented Spanish trail runners, who were clearly relishing the competition from the Canadian duo. I ran at my own pace, feeling the full force of the sun as I passed through villages lined with simple wooden buildings. Friendly locals cheered me on from the relative comfort of shady palm trees, wondering what on earth this woman with bright pink calf guards was doing. It felt amazing to be immersed in this stunning country, but the overwhelming feeling was one of heat.

Unlike before the Marathon des Sables, I hadn't been acclimatising to heat with hot yoga, as work hours were intense. At each of the checkpoints we were reminded by volunteers to drink everything we had left and then refill our bottles. I had a two-litre bladder in a small backpack with a drinking tube, enabling me to have enough water between the checkpoints, before refilling them each time. I didn't feel that thirsty, but my body felt like it was heating from within and I was worried about becoming dehydrated. I was aware that I wanted to push myself, but I also tried to be sensible and slow down as the hours ticked by.

Midway through the day Turbo dropped back from the leading pack of Simon, Salvador and Manu, and I caught up with him near the end of the stage. He was clearly struggling, having gone out too fast. It's always tempting to try and hit a target pace in a race, but conditions such as high wind, heat or humidity can make it too high an effort to keep up for the full course. I tried to think instead about a constant steady effort, so with that in mind I was being more conservative, thinking it was only day one with a long way to go. My steadier pacing paid off and I finished the stage first female in 03:41:32 and seventh overall. The heat had affected me, though, and I could not take advantage of all the food in my drop bag, turning my nose up at all my dehydrated meals. I felt physically unable to eat, which in hindsight hindered my recovery.

At 36km the second day was slightly longer, along mainly flat sandy tracks. We passed through bamboo forest, jungle, dirt roads and flooded fields, the route marked by small flags we had to be alert enough to spot and follow. Children ran by my side through villages wanting high fives and giggled away at the sight of a foreign runner in strange clothing. Given our remote location, we were never too far from the ominous skull and crossbones danger signs for minefields, bitter reminders of the beautiful country's recent history.

That night our camp was within the magnificent grounds of the rarely visited Preah Khan Temple – built in 1131 by King Suryavarman II. I took time to walk slowly around by myself, marvelling at the maze of thousand-year-old carved columns.

The jungle had encroached on the temple in the centuries since it had been abandoned, wrapping itself around the columns and reclaiming the land for itself. I reflected on how fortunate I was to be there, connecting with people, nature and the heart of a beautiful country.

That day I finished first female again in 04:58:54 and still felt I was running well, having settled into the race as usual, my body accepting it needed to get up and run every day. I never felt I was pushing the pace, I just ran consistently and never seemed to slow down. This was despite having to wade through waist-high rivers and navigate claggy muddy trails owing to heavy rainfall the night before. Much of the day I had been running on my own, so it was lovely to catch up with camp mates during the evening and wash off the mud in a nearby river. I was also glad of the luxury of fresh pants and socks in my drop bag to change into at camp. While I loved the simplicity of the carry-everything races like Marathon des Sables and Iceland, I'd felt I proved I could do that and wanted it just to be about the running. But I was aware that things were only going to get tougher.

The next day was a much longer stage, some 62km, first through jungle and then on to the trails, finishing at the incredible Prasat Boeng Mealea Temple, which looks like it has been lifted from an Indiana Jones film set. The conditions were forecast to be more extreme – higher temperatures and even higher humidity – and I was worried about how I'd cope. I was continuing to struggle to take in calories, as my appetite for anything other than sweets had all but disappeared.

However, I wasn't overly concerned about my health; for many runners this was a common occurrence on longer races, especially those in the heat. In the running community, ultramarathons are often described as eating and drinking races. Finishing can depend more on the strength of your stomach than your legs. Apart from the porridge in Morocco, I'd never struggled with eating during a race – getting to eat more than usual was a highlight, especially with the children's party food on offer at many ultras. I often joked my stomach was my strongest muscle, so not being able to eat was a new experience for me.

Everyone was nervous about this long day and, given the length of the route, I was focused on getting it done as quickly as possible to maximise my rest. By this point, though, I was very tired and weak – all because I couldn't stomach food. I remember feeling extremely hot as I gradually made my way through the river crossings and sticky mud, but I kept on moving, overtaking male competitors along the route. I finally crossed the line in 09:41:48 and sank into an unstable plastic chair, exhausted. I tried to tell myself it was supposed to be tough. It was the longest stage after all and the conditions were extreme. Competitors were expected to be on course until midnight. But still something felt very different.

Throughout the stage the humid air had hung around my shoulders like a weighted blanket, making each stride laboured. Just breathing had been difficult. It had been like sucking a thick milkshake through a straw. All day I had struggled to quench my thirst, drinking more and more at each checkpoint, encouraged by volunteers to 'drink up' to ensure I did not become dehydrated. My eyes were struggling to focus – I could make out the stone walls of the ruined temple which surrounded us, but their carved patterns were a blur. Our tents were already set up in neat rows in a clearing and the race crew had started to heat water over a fire. I knew what my next steps should be – find my pack and take it to my shared tent, then prepare my food while I chatted with other runners, sharing stories of the day. This was playing out in my head, but I couldn't physically work out how to start.

The film crew called me over for an interview, but I couldn't move and they had to come to me. Few runners had got back by that point – it seemed the 62km course through the jungle was taking most competitors much longer than expected. Only six runners crossed the line before me and much of the field had slowed to a walk.

'Great job today, Soph. Third female. How was it?'

'It was tough. Really tough. I think I'm in trouble. I feel very dizzy, very dizzy.'

I've been in difficult situations many times before on races – hypothermia, nausea, heatstroke, dehydration. Each time I was able to analyse my symptoms, understand what had happened and treat myself accordingly. But right at that moment I wasn't able to understand what was happening. I was confused, my mental capacity to make sense of things had drained away and I didn't know why but I was truly scared. By now the film crew and I knew each other well. They'd seen me hypothermic in Iceland and they too sensed something was different this time. They called the medics over to assess my condition as I lay on the temple steps, completely vacant. I was led to my tent and helped to lie down. I started throwing up and was extremely disoriented, as if someone else had taken over my body. With my eyes glazed over I lay in a huddle as the medics dispensed two IV bags into my veins and covered me with a foil blanket.

Krasse, my new Bulgarian friend, stayed by my side all evening, trying to get me to eat more and recover, but the next morning I felt even worse. I remained confused and was finding it difficult to balance my body as I walked, swaying side to side. Behind the scenes race director Stefan Betzelt had been consulting with my friends Simon, Turbo and Krasse, as well as the medics Florian and Achim, over my condition. They decided they needed to pull me from the race. I had also come to the same conclusion, and instead of a 30km run along dusty roads and muddy jungle footpaths I was driven to the next campsite at Phnom Kulen Waterfalls to await the rest of the runners. The plan was for me to rejoin the race the next day if I felt better, so I was able to experience the magnificent Angkor Wat temple finale, despite not being officially in the race.

As I entered the next campsite, I was relieved to see it surrounded by several raised wooden platforms, about three metres across, with shaded tops made of thatch. It looked like the perfect location for a spa. I lay down on the wooden slats and watched the crew set up the tents around me. I don't remember much about the day except the moment a tiny kitten came and sat with me as I rested and tried to recover my senses.

I have no memory of what happened next, but it was recorded by the film crew and I have watched it back on screen many times since. It makes for truly horrifying viewing. That afternoon I got up to walk around camp and welcome the runners as they began to arrive, but I suddenly collapsed and went into cardiac arrest. The medics grabbed the defibrillator and revived me. I was alive – but only just. I was unconscious with one side of my face paralysed, as if I'd had a stroke. On watching the film I can hear one of the medics saying, 'She's dying, she's nearly dead.' It turned out that I had drunk too much water and, as I had not eaten enough salt, my salt levels had been diluted by all the fluid in my body. This had caused severe hyponatremia and a cerebral oedema – meaning my brain was swollen. The normal sodium level in the body is 130mg/l. Severe effects occur below 120. Mine had fallen to just 108. And I was in a remote location in the Cambodian jungle.

Stefan immediately called a helicopter to take me to a hospital in Siem Reap, the nearest town, which was 50km away. As the red helicopter swept into camp 16 minutes later the remaining competitors were left shellshocked. It had all happened so quickly. The runners were told that I was in a 'more than critical' condition and the two medics were accompanying me to hospital. Once I arrived at Angkor International Hospital the emergency doctors decided they needed to drill a hole in my skull to reduce the pressure from my swollen brain. But that could only be done in a more specialist hospital. So Stefan chartered a second helicopter to take me 400km to Bangkok in Thailand. He put the helicopter fees on his own credit card without checking I had medical insurance (I did), knowing any delay would worsen my chances of survival. I'll always be deeply grateful to him. His quick thinking undoubtedly saved my life.

By this point, my mother, brother Adam and John were on a plane to Bangkok, with my father staying at home to manage logistics. I cannot imagine the torment in their minds as they flew – not knowing what they would find when they landed – while I lay in a coma, fighting for my life. My brother, who is in the army, had been through incredibly stressful life or death situations before and was trained for extreme events. He was the person most able to detach himself and stay focused on what needed doing.

Their tickets were all to Siem Reap – to the first hospital I was sent to – and I was still there when they took off from Heathrow. Luckily, they were flying via Bangkok first, so, having been given an update, they disembarked and came straight to the hospital. I was in intensive care by the time they arrived and still in a coma, but I was alive. My mum slumped to the floor in shock when she first caught sight of me wired up to a series of beeping machines. Nothing can prepare you for seeing your child in serious peril. John was in a daze, later describing the situation as a surreal and distressing experience from out of the blue. Anxiously my family waited by my bedside, and around 36 hours after I fell unconscious, I started to come round. My family were prepared for the worst. There was no guarantee what mental state I would be in. Few people who have sodium levels that low survive, never mind recover.

As I came to my senses I realised I had been bundled into a helicopter and taken to hospital. I was relieved to see John, my brother and my mum, but one look at their faces made me realise how close to death I had been. As the hours went by I became more alert, sending Facebook messages and emails to Stefan asking him how to repay him. I somehow managed to type 'in bangkok hospital recovering from race' on Facebook less than 12 hours after I came round. The following day I uploaded another quick post warning everyone about the limited strength of standard electrolyte tablets. I remember my strong sense of injustice and desire to ensure that no one would ever make the same mistake.

Back at the race Stefan had 'neutralised' the fifth stage, allowing everyone to walk or run a shorter distance, before racing the final stage to Angkor Wat the day after. He handled the situation perfectly – allowing runners to complete the course, but respecting the conditions and the safety. Meanwhile, at the hospital, it started to emerge that I had no belongings. My evacuation out of the jungle had been so rapid that all I had with me was my passport. My mum scrambled around trying to find me clothes, but all she could find was a pair of pink maternity leggings from the hospital shop.

By day four post collapse I was pleading with the doctor to discharge me. It was not going to happen. The eighth drip had just been hooked up to my arm and my CAT scan still made me look like a dead person. Fortunately, they moved me out of intensive care, to a room with a view at the top of the hospital. By now I was eating well and my spirits definitely lifted when my brother appeared with a batch of Dunkin' Donuts which I eagerly devoured. Simon and Turbo even came to visit on their way back to Canada, giving me a further boost and bringing my bag, as well as an Indiana Jones t-shirt, which hung off my gaunt frame. Two days later, and just six days after I collapsed, I found myself homeward bound: I was upgraded for medical reasons to business class, drinking champagne. I had never been so relieved to have corporate health insurance.

No one knows why I recovered when so many others don't, but the doctors surmised that my high fitness levels must have played a part. While being an endurance runner got me into this situation, it also probably got me out of it alive and roughly in one piece. But I was not unaffected. I had limited short-term memory for many weeks. At the end of a conversation, I often forgot what had just been said. But, somehow, I went straight back to work, not even taking an additional day off beyond the holiday I had booked for the race itself. I was chief financial officer of an international marketing agency and we were in the midst of a restructure. I'd been away less than two weeks, but urgent requests were coming in from all over the world that needed my attention, and the chairman and CEO put pressure on me to come to the office and deal with them. I had clearly been through a trauma and still needed to recover, yet the world continued to spin as if nothing had happened.

My doctor happened to be friends with the company chairman and spoke to him, imploring him to let me rest, but not once was I told to go home. If this happened now, I would not hesitate to put my health first, just as I would do for anyone working for me; but in that moment I didn't yet have the confidence and the sense of my true priorities to do so. I felt a huge sense of guilt for putting my family through so much distress, but I struggled to reconcile that genuine guilt with the fact that I had not knowingly put myself at risk. I had not been illegally base jumping off a building or doing some other, high-risk daredevil stunt. In fact, it was my very focus on being sensible and drinking water that had caused the problem. I wasn't fully aware of the risks of hyponatremia, nor the high level of salt in my sweat. I only discovered this later through a specialised test, which revealed I was at a higher risk than others. I was encouraged to keep drinking by the race volunteers and although, unlike in the Marathon des Sables, salt tablets were not handed out I had brought my own. However, I was relying on a brand that turned out to be insufficient in strength for me, and I'd forgotten to take them regularly anyway.

Following the trauma of Cambodia I felt an intense pressure from friends, family and colleagues to just stop running, as if running was a dangerous activity, with the risks outweighing the benefits. Looking back it reminds me of the pressure society puts on pregnant women to sit on the couch and eat cake rather than 'risk the baby' through movement.

At no point did I consider giving up running as an option. I loved it too much and I reasoned to myself that these risks were all controllable in the future. Why should I give up the running adventures that I loved? But that's not to say I didn't struggle after the event. Looking for answers I turned to one of my tent mates from the Marathon des Sables: Ian the psychologist. We'd spoken at length during the race about the mental makeup of those of us who undertook these challenges, and our many different reasons for attempting them. In the midst of such an extreme race, with all luxuries stripped away and our bodies under constant duress, there is no possibility of faking anything – we had no energy to pretend to be anything other than our core self. Our tent of eight strangers had bonded strongly that week, and I left feeling my tent mates were amongst a minority of my friends who truly knew the real me, warts and all. I had a feeling Ian might be able to help me think through my situation, and find a path out of the guilt and confusion that was enclosing me.

With Ian's help I was able, for the first time, to reflect on a future I might never have had; a future for my family without me. One seemingly logical outcome to this 'near-death' experience might have been that John and I started living every day for itself, less mindful of any longer-term consequences for our health, finances and more. And in a way for a while we did. It was close to Christmas, but even so we were indulging more than usual. We accepted every party invitation and stayed out until the early hours. We bought each other more gifts and started to plan adventure holidays for the coming year. But what Ian helped me do was unravel the puzzles in my mind, and understand how I could move forwards and learn from my experience.

My mental turmoil wasn't just due to the physical experience in Cambodia and my feelings of guilt afterwards. It was because, having been made acutely aware of my own mortality, I had begun to question the meaning and direction of my life. Plunging straight back into the commercial rat race after such a life-changing experience felt like hitting a wall. Everything seemed so superficial and devoid of value. I felt I shouldn't even be there, not fit and healthy anyway. And yet I was. Questions filled my mind. Is this it? Where is my path taking me? Will it lead me somewhere I even want to be? I imagined pressing fast-forward on my life, visualising the future. Where do I actually want to be and what path will take me there?

Having to contemplate my life coming to a full stop, and then picturing the future for my family without me, allowed me for the first time to think freely and imagine the future I really wanted – not the life that I'd assumed I wanted, the one I felt society had pressured me into as I rose quickly through my career, smashing ceilings with my red-soled stilettos. I quickly realised that so many of the career goals I had set myself played very little part in the future I longed for and, in many ways, achieving those goals made that future less likely. When asked 'what really matters to you?' the answer for most of us is our family and friends, our health and security. Despite that, I realised I and almost everyone around me were living lives with different priorities. I drew pie charts of what mattered to me and where I spent my time and energy. The two were vastly different. This made me realise I was getting it so wrong.

I was working long hours and spending much of my time travelling. My parents were less than two hours away from my London home, but I rarely visited without an 'official' reason to do so like a birthday or mothers' day. I spent more of my social time with work colleagues than my long-term friends – those who would be there for me long after I inevitably changed jobs – and I'd barely even considered having our own family. My trajectory was to be CFO of a FTSE 100 company, to rapidly ascend the career ladder, even if it meant sacrificing time with friends and family. That's what I thought I should do. That's what achievement meant. If I chose not to I would be 'wasting' my education, my hard work over the past years. Success was status, money, power.

I'd never known anything different, but I no longer wanted this. The future I now visualised had more time for me; time to spend with the people I loved, rather than slaving away for a workplace that gave no consideration to my physical or mental health. I wanted my own family and to have meaning in my life, which positively impacted those around me. In Cambodia I'd been helped and saved by others, and I understood first-hand the significant power of the kindness of strangers. I wanted to be the person that could make a positive difference to someone else's life. Private equity was all about shutting things down, selling people out, closing jobs – making profit at any cost. Deep down I felt this wasn't right, and I yearned to do something purposeful. Nothing made sense to me anymore. I was lost and knew things had to dramatically change.

For the first time it became clear that not only did I truly want to be a mother, I wanted to do it sooner rather than later. While I found it hard to imagine choosing to be neck-deep in nappies (at my niece's christening I refused to hold her for fear she would vomit all over my silver Stella McCartney suit), I couldn't detach myself from the desire to create my own family with John.

As my mind unwound itself from the trauma, my true definition of what success and happiness looked like became stronger, and I started to analyse others' lives to gain insight into what might work for us. John and I had met as interns at an investment bank, working in mergers and acquisitions. We had both joined after university yet barely saw one another, as we worked late into the evening, most weekends and sometimes even overnight. There was no point in making weekend plans together as they were sure to be cancelled by yet another 'important' meeting that needed to be prepared for, which was itself often cancelled at short notice. We looked towards the senior bankers as a vision of what our future would look like if we succeeded in climbing the ladder.

They mostly had families, and children they rarely saw for bedtime and holidays that were interrupted daily with long calls with clients. This was the definition of success – rising up the ladder, earning high salaries, bonuses and 'prestige'. But what for? To afford central London housing, private schooling, designer clothes and luxury holidays – but at the expense of control over their lives and precious time with their young children. Something they would never be able to get back later in their lives, once they had made the financial fortunes they prioritised. It was a future I realised I didn't want.

Yet it was happening all around us. We began to see the negative effects amongst our own friends of the mismatch between their stated priorities and where they spent their time. Some were working so many hours, intent on progressing in their career and making more money to support their family, that they neglected the relationships that truly mattered, which then fell apart. Many of my girlfriends in similar careers were well into their thirties and were too busy to meet a life partner and start a family.

My experience in Cambodia allowed us to think much more clearly about what really mattered, and how each part of our life fitted together. Focusing on the future vision made those important short- or medium-term decisions easier to make, even if they went against maximising short-term gains.

Soon after my return from Cambodia, we started trying for a family. And when I finally became pregnant almost a year later, and realised that the toxic air pollution along my walking commute was harming my unborn son, I left my fast-track finance career to co-found a company to find the solution. I had been working with start-up companies on the side for many years as an outlet for my entrepreneurial spirit. When I met someone willing to invest in my idea I immediately knew I had to take the leap. Without that new clarity of thought I would never have taken the decision to do so – it would have seemed like too much of a risk – but I now knew I wasn't heading in the right direction. My vision of where I wanted to go – where we as a family wanted to go – had radically changed.

Perhaps what Cambodia did most of all was make me want to truly live my life to the full – with no regrets. Not living just for each day itself, in case there would not be another, but for my overall life and happiness. Every now and then I think of where my old paths might have led – seeing friends and former colleagues excel in those careers, increasing their salary year by year. But instead of the jealousy I may once have felt, I allow myself to imagine those paths, and what I would lose from my life today had I followed them. I will never regret working fewer hours in an office and spending more time with my children. I will never regret spending time with my parents or investing in relationships with my friends. I will never regret working for positive social impact instead of working to increase profits at a faceless company.

While I was heartbroken for my family at what had happened in Cambodia and the pain it had caused those around me, ultimately it was a transformational experience that had become a catalyst for positive change. It enabled me to reframe everything in my life and question where I was headed. I had a second chance and seized the moment. There was no looking back – no regrets, just the road ahead.

Coda: Never regret

Life is unpredictable and sometimes it takes a moment of crisis to see what truly matters. Facing the possibility of death made me realise that success isn't about titles or material gains, but about time, relationships and living with purpose. Fear of change can keep us trapped in a path that doesn't serve us, but we always have the power to reassess, to shift direction and to choose a life that aligns with our values. Don't wait for a wake-up call – take control now. Live boldly, love deeply and make decisions that lead to a life without regrets.

4
PRESS RESET

Stage racing in Nepal, Iceland and Bhutan

'You shouldn't be doing this anymore. It's far too dangerous. Look what happened last time.' My family were frightened. My near-death experience in Cambodia had reverberated painfully around those closest to me, and understandably they were concerned for my safety. But several months had passed and I was fully recovered, raring to go once more. I couldn't just sit on the sofa and relax. I respected how terrified my family were, but the right answer wasn't to stop. It was to work out what had happened and take control.

A specialist sweat test had given me the understanding I needed. Working out how much sodium I sweated out per litre of water meant I knew exactly how much to replenish. My body needed more than four times the amount of sodium (1g of salt is about 400mg of sodium) I had been taking in Cambodia (when I remembered the electrolyte tablets), and this was a straightforward problem to fix. I needed 1000mg of sodium per litre of water. I knew my body didn't cope well in hot humid conditions, but there were plenty of other climates it could tolerate. With no race on the calendar I felt empty and had nothing to look forward to. It wasn't about testing my limits anymore – I knew I could complete these races – but it was a desperate yearning for connection and escape. Slipping into a coma had ripped this experience away and my memories of Cambodia were patchy at best. I needed another adventure, both for my mental health and to have closure on Cambodia.

Stage racing had been a huge part of my life since Marathon des Sables, and for the past two and half years it had been my only form of escapism. I'd sit in the office dreaming ahead to the next adventure. Post-Cambodia I found myself reflecting back on my pursuits overseas. Exploring remote places I would never normally have had access to was a self-affirming experience. I felt connected with the landscape, the local communities and most of all my fellow runners. At every race there was a self-selected bunch of people who loved the outdoors and the simple life, who were willing to push themselves through adversity. There were no preconceptions about who you were, what you did or where you went to university. It was the antithesis of working in finance, where you had to dress a certain way, speak and act correctly and be from the right background (apart from a small minority like John and I). Out in the middle of nowhere it was all about how you supported and interacted with others, and the sense of shared experience. Lifelong friendships were made on the trails and I forged bonds with the most incredible people. For those few days we were a family, with the fastest runners all pitching in to support the slowest. We helped others however we could, sharing kit, advice and fuel to ensure everyone had the best chance of achieving their goal. We stayed up late each day to clap in the final finisher. We worked as a team and created a home wherever we ran.

This was the polar opposite of the world of triathlon, which in my late twenties I had briefly dabbled in. While I was riding the high of completing Marathon des Sables, John had been Lycra-deep into the world of multi-discipline sport. During a holiday in Nicaragua, he gave me a long speech over dinner about the lengthy hours of training required in the lead-up to his Ironman challenge. He was taking it very seriously and implied that it was going to be a lot harder than my running training. I had to be understanding, he said, and accept that his weekends would be taken up with running, swimming and cycling. I'm not quite sure what got into me (though it may have been the second – or third – glass of wine), but I thought to myself *how hard can it be?* John got up to go to the toilet and by the time he returned I'd signed myself up for Ironman Switzerland. 'But Sophie, you can barely swim and you never ride your bike,' was his incredulous response.

He was absolutely correct. I could only swim 25 metres without getting out of breath, and when riding a bike, I couldn't even take my left hand off the handlebars to indicate (I still wobble when I do). However, as usual the drive to prove myself capable was stronger than my common sense. And anyway, I had nine months to learn how to swim 3.6km and cycle 180km; and the marathon at the end would be something to look forward to.

With an Ironman on the horizon, John and I threw ourselves into the weekend-warrior lifestyle, working long hours all week and training hard all weekend. Saturday morning was a double spin class followed by a swim with a longish run on Sundays. I did an immersive swimming course over a weekend, which stopped me panicking in the water, and then gradually built up my swimming stamina. Although I never seemed to get faster, I was finally convinced I could make it round without drowning. I never felt that comfortable on a bike, especially with my hands on the drop bars, away from the brakes, but I was confident I could go fast enough with my endurance engine to make it around. Looking at the cut-offs they allowed six hours for the final marathon. At least that part would be easy.

I'd DNF'd a training triathlon when my chain broke and couldn't be repaired, so Ironman Switzerland was my first chance to finish one. Sadly, it was not to be the experience I'd hoped for. This was 2011 and before the time of rolling starts. Thousands of people entered the water at once, creating a seafood soup of thrashing limbs. As I stood at the mass start I was overrun with a sense of terror. Rather than being excited to race, I feared entering the dark water. Holding back, I entered at the last minute, right at the back of the pack. Regrettably, the cautious approach was all in vain. Within seconds I had competitors swimming over the top of me, pushing me towards the bottom of the lake to gain extra seconds. Minutes later one of my fillings was knocked out by a thundering punch, leading to an expensive Swiss dentistry bill. When I finally left the water 96 minutes later, I found myself in a maelstrom of bicycles with men blocking me from overtaking. I had still not mastered the art of lifting one hand from the bars, so each time I wanted water I had to grind to a complete stop. It was not the most efficient technique in the world. Despite this, I loved the uphill stretches and steep climbs passing through a gauntlet of cowbells and cheers.

Once I reached the final marathon running stage I was able to relax a little, enjoying the sense of relative security from running on tarmac. As I nipped along the road, I passed John, who by this point was clearly suffering in the heat, which was always his nemesis. I checked he was OK before pushing on, finishing ahead of him.

My overall impression of the race was far from glowing. In fact, I tried to wipe most of it from my memory. It was busy, masculine and unfriendly. No-one chatted to each other and there was zero camaraderie. Everyone was purely focused on their own race, crunching numbers and monitoring splits. There was a huge amount of peacocking with flashy £10,000 cow print bikes on display and the latest tech wizardry wetsuits. And most sad of all? The checkpoints did not have cake. Or Haribo. This was clearly not my kind of race.

Although it was entirely my fault I had signed up for Switzerland, in the spirit of retaliation I registered John for a weeklong Racing the Planet stage race in Nepal, selling it as a 'trekking holiday'. It was time he entered my world, so three months after the horror of Ironman we found ourselves in a tiny propeller plane hurtling through the mountains towards Pokhara. This was more like it. Along with 213 runners from 42 countries, we would cover approximately 220km in seven days over rough terrain, with only a tent and water provided. Some days we would be climbing 3000m, but with my hiking background and logistical experience from Marathon des Sables this felt exactly in my wheelhouse. What I hadn't anticipated was sickness. On the eve of our departure around 70 of the runners – including me – came down with food poisoning from the hotel buffet. I was reduced to a stunned, nauseous heap in my tent, my stomach twisting so fiercely I wondered if I'd even start. For the first few days I was completely wiped out, John hauling me up and down the steep rocky trails, pausing to admire the majestic mountains while I emptied my stomach yet again. When I couldn't keep any other food down, in a moment of true sacrifice he gave me his beloved wine gums. I'd definitely married the right man.

Unfortunately, the sickness spread through the camp, taking with it every last piece of toilet paper. Despite the grimness of the situation, the camaraderie amongst the runners was infectious and John understood for the first time what was so special about these races. The people, their generosity and their humour was so incredibly heartwarming, especially when juxtaposed against the commerciality of the race itself. At every turn we felt manipulated by the organisers who saw us as marketing fodder. They wanted us to destroy all our upper body kit by sewing on patches with their logo, the idea being that it would be great for their video footage. I refused to do it to my waterproof jacket and stuck it on with sticky tape instead which was very much against the ridiculous 'rules'.

Thankfully, the runners around us did a great job of rallying together and providing distraction against a backdrop of diarrhoea and vomiting. We chatted late into each evening around the campfire, expertly attended to by Canadians. My spirits were continually uplifted by a team of three hilarious Irish guys sharing our tent. One of them was reading a book called *Watching the English* about the quirks and foibles of English people. Every time he read a page, he ripped it out to use it as toilet paper. It was such an on-the-nose gesture for an Irishman to be wiping his arse on a book about the English that it tickled us for days. It wasn't until the final day – buoyed by pizza from a local teahouse — that I was finally able to run. But it didn't matter. The whole time I had focused on moving with purpose, absorbing the dramatic surroundings and warmly greeting locals with a colloquial 'Namaste'. There was no hurry, no competition, just adventure. Instead of conversations about climbing the career ladder, we shared our favourite races and discussed bucket list challenges. It was the first time I heard people talking about 100-milers and, as is the danger on these kinds of events, I started pondering what I should do next. A 100-mile race in the UK sounded feasible, given the cut-offs were often 30 hours, which was a walking pace. I had already completed a few 50-mile races, and had seen how many people simply hiked the whole course in Nepal. I also had the experience of moving through the night in the Marathon des Sables, which gave me the confidence to tackle a 30-hour race. A plan started to hatch.

I left Nepal lighter in body and mind. I had lost weight from the sickness — so much so that I thought about the need to put on weight for the first time in my life — but more positively my mind felt replenished. My faith in humanity had been restored. Not everyone was fighting to compete. Many were simply along for the ride, keen to forge connections and have a great time while doing it. I couldn't wait for the next adventure.

By now I well and truly had the ultramarathon bug. Over the next year I logged eight of them, including my first 100-mile race. In hindsight it was a crazy number of ultras, but I was childfree and impatient to soak up every experience. The Centurion Thames Path 100 was my gateway to 24-hour racing. It was a 100-mile race along the banks of the River Thames, starting in Richmond and ending in Oxford. Restricted to 300 competitors — which was a relatively large number for this distance, at the time — it mostly attracted runners from the UK. To qualify for entry, you had to have completed a race of at least 50 miles within 15 hours. It was a moderately competitive race owing to its strict 29 hour cut off time, but the terrain was flat and unchallenging. Drop bags with spare clothing and food were allowed at miles 51 and 71, pacers were allowed for the final 41 miles, and support crew were permitted at designated spots enroute. The 12 aid stations were well stocked with sweet and savoury snacks, making the race accessible to first timers as well as those fighting for a podium position.

Little did I know that this was the foundation for future World Championships and record attempts. Instead, I treated it like a 50-mile race with some hiking tacked on. My strategy was to run as far as I could then switch to run-walking. I never dreamed I would finish in under 24 hours, I was just curious about the experience. It went something like this: run for 50 miles then do a 10-minute run followed by a two-minute walk. As time ticked by, this dropped to an eight-minute run followed by a two-minute walk, and so on. My brother Adam crewed me while John joined me as a pacer with 40 miles to go, managing the walk breaks on his watch to save my mental energy. He was also a safety net as I got increasingly tired, and he made sure I didn't stumble into the river. With 30 miles to go, it got to the point where I screamed at him, 'I'm not running anymore!' (I think there might have been a swear word or two in there as well). Calm as ever, he told me to fast-hike it out, which I did. As I would later discover, the problem with a flat race like this was having no natural place to slow down to walk and eat, like you would on a mountainous race during a climb, so chunking it up and deciding when to eat was in some ways more difficult.

Using my Nordic walking poles, I marched through the mud to the finish in 23 hours, 11 minutes. A particularly poignant moment was turning onto a final bend and catching sight of the Christ Church boat house I used to row from while at Oxford University. I realised I had just run 100 miles to that boat house, when a few years earlier I couldn't even run the one mile to it from my university accommodation. I had come a long way literally and metaphorically.

We'd been moving through a March snow storm and the race was called off shortly after I finished. I was delighted at my time and pleased to tick off a 100-miler in one piece, but it still didn't scratch my underlying itch. I still yearned for the overseas experience, exploring somewhere new. My calendar became a series of races planned around wherever my job took me next. I was still working as chief financial officer for the global marketing agency with 14 markets across the world, so international travel was mandatory. I tried to visit every market at least once every couple of years and tie it in with a personal trip. During the Lions Rugby Tour in Australia, I 'just so happened' to need to be Down Under for work. When I needed to travel to South Africa I made sure it was during the week of Comrades, the world's oldest ultramarathon. Luckily, I had a qualifying marathon time from my Ironman race, so it did come in useful after all. In fact, John managed to convince me to sign up for another triathlon in the French city of Vichy. It was another unpleasant encounter, but it was a sacrifice I was willing to take in return for us doing another stage race together. John has requested I add here that he was faster than me this time, although it was reduced to a 70.3, or 'half Ironman' the night before with temperatures reaching 40 degrees, so my Ironman record against him is intact.

Having no children meant we were pretty flexible and could race as much as work allowed. It was easy to drop everything and go away even at short notice, and our annual leave was used up on racing 'holidays'. We were fortunate enough to have the finances to pay for these experiences; race fees often reach several hundred – or even thousand - pounds each, plus the cost of travel, accommodation, food and kit. Often we were the youngest participants, as these challenges typically attracted older individuals with more disposable income and free time. All our holiday budget was put towards races, and we were always straight back at our desks with battered bodies and blistered feet as soon as the race was over. Walking to the tube was our recovery. But we didn't want the thrill to end. Next stop: Iceland.

Beginning atop a glittering glacier in Vatnajökull National Park, the Fire and Ice six-day footrace swept across 250km of raw wilderness stretching all the way to the crashing northern shores.

Compared to the over-the-top commercial circus of the Nepal race – where sending an email a day cost $50 and we were walking ad billboards – the stripped-back scale felt like a breath of fresh air. And I felt secure knowing my additional warm clothing was tucked safely away in the emergency cold weather bag, ready for the crew to hand over at the first sign of trouble which, of course, came swiftly.

As with most multi-day events, the course carved through landscapes that seemed plucked from fantasy. The race organisers made every effort to take us to remote, untouched areas that the normal traveller could not reach without support. One dawn we sprinted across lush, emerald plains; by the next dusk we found ourselves in a rocky lunar wasteland – an actual astronaut training ground – where not a soul or signpost dotted the horizon. It was one surprise after another. At twilight, during the middle of the race, we were surprised by the crew who led our weary legs to a steaming hot spring, where we sank into mineral-rich waters beneath a canopy of stars.

Each day, as John and I ran in silent unison, something extraordinary would rise up: jagged lava fields, ancient rock formations and, most unforgettable of all, the thunderous Dettifoss Waterfall – its raw power immortalised in the Ridley Scott film *Prometheus*. I literally skidded to a halt, spellbound by the unwavering might and roar. Moving through untamed Iceland felt like a privilege: I was both spectator and participant in nature's grand theatre, marvelling at its soaring beauty and unforgiving ferocity, every stride reminding me of the planet's majesty and brutality. I had never felt more alive.

It wasn't long before I sampled the brute force of nature first hand, though. Despite the race taking place in the middle of the Icelandic summer, on day three we were hit with unexpected snowstorms. The bleak grey landscape meant we had no place to hide from the 95km/h winds, and each step was a soul-sucking trudge through freezing sludge. As the wind tore at our bodies John and I ran head-down, staring at our frozen feet, protecting our eyes from the driving snow. With temperatures below zero

I was on the verge of hypothermia, my body temperature dropping to unsafe levels. My lips were frozen as I stumbled into the last checkpoint, mumbling to the race crew that I was unable to feel anything. By that point we were walking and I was desperate to run to generate some body heat, but John was in a lot of pain, struggling with an injured Achilles which he'd picked up the day before. Crossing a frozen river near the start of the day had numbed his lower leg, but once this wore off he was in agony.

As I sat crying in the back of the crew car at the aid station drinking hot tea, I made the difficult decision to leave John behind. The camera team – primarily there to film the Canadian duo, Simon Donato and Paul Trebilcock, known as 'Turbo' (filming *Boundless*, a global adventure race series) – captured me whispering through frozen lips, 'I can't walk. It's too cold. I need to run.' John, kindly, but with a slight reluctance in his eyes, told me to go. This loving gesture was captured in the final cut of the *Boundless* episode. The film crew were following Simon and Turbo but along the way captured stories of other competitors, and they seemed particularly interested in the couple dynamic between me and John (and I was one of only two women in the race). Despite feeling guilty leaving him behind, I ran the last 10k stretch to the finish line and anxiously waited for John to arrive. A wave of relief washed over me as he appeared through the snow and I immediately started apologising for sprinting ahead. The camera crew also captured all of this on film, which apparently made for great television. It was my first time in front of the camera and the producers were excited about the impact that I might have on female viewers; they seemed to like me being so open and honest about the challenges I was facing, but also making them seem attainable.

Once more the kindness of strangers left its indelible mark on me during our Nordic expedition. Local Icelanders came out to run stages of the race alongside the competitors and at one point one of these locals, who worked as a shepherd, saved me from extreme hunger when he snuck me a handful of mini-Snickers bars. I was absolutely ravenous for the whole race as I wasn't able to carry the weight of enough calories, but the locals could pop home each night to resupply as they weren't official competitors. The minimum requirement was 2000 calories per day – which I could just about manage to carry – but I was burning two or three times this. As part of the race rules, you were only supposed to eat what you could carry, and were not allowed to be crewed. But there were no rules on being supported by other participants and I will be eternally grateful to the man who handed me those bars of peanuty goodness.

Each night John and I plus a handful of runners camped under the stars, in tents provided by the race. It was a tiny event with around 20 international runners in a location inaccessible by anything other than a four-wheel drive. We had remarkable access to a location where there was nothing more than the odd shepherd's hut. We carried all of our gear except for tents, hot water and emergency warm clothes bags. These were diligently couriered by the race crew in the back of a series of 4x4s. As the week wore on, I learnt about Icelandic culture and became aware of its gender parity. Decades earlier women had gone on strike to demand equal pay and more support from men in the home. The political movement had changed society, making Iceland the most equal country for women on earth. Armed with this knowledge, it felt like the ideal country to be racing in when I crossed the finish first female.

But it wasn't about the winning. That week everyone had been through their own personal journey and there was an overwhelming sense that we had been through it together. This companionship was sealed at the crazy afterparty as we were driven in a limousine to a nightclub in a town called Akureyri. Ending on a runner's high we stuffed our faces with food, downed shots of Black Death (the Icelandic national spirit), and danced the night away as a final celebration of togetherness. It was no surprise that four months later I found myself chasing these same connections, only this time in Cambodia. The lure of the stage race held me in its tight grip.

Returning from Cambodia, I had nothing booked. The emptiness was killing me. I was fit and healthy again, but I had a stage-race-sized gap in my life. I felt like the thing I loved most had been ripped away from me. While other members of my family were still gravely concerned, John understood that I now had a better grasp on my physiology than ever before. I planned metic-ulously, read all the literature and plotted all the variables. John also knew I was only truly happy when I had something to train for. Preventing me from racing would ultimately be more detrimental to my mental health than any of the risks involved in taking part.

I needed to press reset on my Cambodia experience and start over, reconnecting with many of the runners and crew I had met in Southeast Asia. Global Limits had a series of races and many of the participants ticked them off one by one. I knew if I went to Bhutan I would be seeing many familiar faces again – including Stefan, the race director. They had been deeply affected when I suddenly fell into a coma right in front of their eyes, and I needed to show them I had come back stronger and was ready for closure. I knew many of them would be racing in Bhutan and I was especially keen to see Edda Bauer, an incredible German runner. She was born in 1944 and started ultrarunning in her sixties. She was an inspiring force of nature and I hoped that in later life I could be like her.

Nervously emailing Stefan I asked if I could come to his next race in Bhutan. He deferred to Jeremy, the medical direc-tor, who said that if I promised not to 'race', I was welcome. Coincidentally, I needed to travel to India that year, because my firm was looking at buying a company there. Aligning my work and hobby once more, I set up meetings in Bangalore for the post-race week. I was heading back out for another adven-ture armed with a bespoke sodium and hydration plan, just six months after waking from a coma.

I arrived in the Bhutan capital Thimphu bleary-eyed after a long flight from London, half-wondering if I was doing the right thing, but the moment I caught sight of my friends a wave of relief washed over me. We crashed into each other with squishy hugs that felt like coming home. All my nervousness – Would I be fit enough? Would my legs remember how to climb? How would the altitude affect me? – simply melted away. I'd promised myself a conservative race strategy: go slow, eat often, rest hard and keep well within my means. There would be six stages and 200km to cover, but with nightly access to my drop bag full of food I could afford to carry only light trail snacks, a large hand-ful of salt tabs and an appetite for adventure.

On the Friday morning we were whisked off to explore Thimphu's cultural treasures. The National Memorial Chorten stood immense and white-washed against a cobalt sky, its golden spires shining in the brazen sunlight. Inside, incense curls drifted up around gilded statues and monks' chanting echoed through the hush. I traced the ancient murals with my eyes and savoured the scent of butter lamps. While Nepal had been a heady rush of noisy crowded streets, Bhutan by comparison was infused with an ethereal calm. It was the perfect soothing atmosphere to mentally prepare for the days ahead. I was exactly where I needed to be.

The first day began under an emotional chorus of voices at Punakha Dzong. Hundreds of school children with bright eyes lined up to sing Bhutan's national anthem under the watch-ful eye of the district governor. It was the first international race ever to be held in the country, with 36 runners represent-ing 16 nations. Setting off on the 30km stage, a band of giddy kids accompanied us through the start line before peeling off to return to the classroom. The route travelled along a beautiful, lush valley flanked either side by rolling hills covered in dense woodland. The mild temperature (around 18 degrees Celsius) was perfect for running and I soon found myself in step with Danish runner Zenia Inselmann, the woman in the lead. Before long we arrived at Bhutan's longest suspension bridge, where I shuffled across the swinging wooden slats, my calves quiver-ing with nerves. Settling into a steady jog, Zenia and I stuck together for the rest of the day, both glad of the company.

This remained our formation for the entirety of the race. When Zenia was struggling on the 1700m climb up Sinchula Pass on day two I remained by her side and talked her through. During stage three the roles were reversed and Zenia supported me as my energy dissipated. There was never any question of us racing one another. We were simply enjoying being together and sharing the experience. We discussed how we were feeling and took time to stop together at the prayer wheels on the roadside. We took turns to spin the wheels, reflecting on our journey and what lay ahead.

Despite my waning energy, day three was the highlight of the week as a 1000m climb delivered us to Phajoding Monastery. Flags snapped in the mountain breeze as we entered one of the most decorated monasteries in Bhutan, but it wasn't the holy relics that left their mark on my memory. Instead, it was the young, orphaned monks' holy dedication to football. The walls of the living quarters were plastered with newspaper cuttings of football matches, and when I got roped into helping with some English homework, the exercise was filling in the blanks of the lyrics to the Liverpool FC song 'You'll Never Walk Alone'. It seemed such a juxtaposition. Here we sat in the holiest of places, perched in the mountains at 3600m altitude, and all these devout child monks were obsessed with European football.

That evening we booted balls across the courtyard with the resident monks – my football skills embarrassingly sub-par, yet the laughter echoed higher than the peaks. I kicked the ball around a few times, but afraid of letting the team down (as well as of injury) I quickly subbed myself out – a wise move as moments later an older runner injured their leg. Fortunately for him I had packed spare hiking poles, as he needed them for the steep descent through the forest the following day.

The 37km stage crisscrossed up and down the Pumula Pass before it finally crossed some paddy fields. The camp was set up at a local farmhouse where we were able to relieve our aching muscles in a traditional hot stone bath – the ideal recovery before the 52km long stage day.

By this point I had done enough multi-day races to recognise that each one had a longer stage, usually on the penultimate day. This was a little trickier to pull off in the Bhutanese foothills where there were limited places to camp, and limited flattish ground where distance came easier. To make it a long enough distance, the course looped around the airport in the Paro Valley through narrow paddy field tracks. I was constantly balancing and counterbalancing as I navigated the thin paths of mud through flooded fields. At one point I kept going wrong, losing the tracks which were marked with ribbons on sticks. Instead, I kept catching sight of girls with ribbons in their hair, leading to much confusion. Thankfully the local farmers pointed me in the right direction and eventually I found my way, finishing at the ruins of Drukgyal Dzong bathed in golden evening sunlight.

The final day did not disappoint. It was just 14km, but it wound up the mountainside with a heart-pounding 4km climb to Paro Taktsang, which sat at 3100m above sea level. The monastery, also known as Tiger's Nest and made famous in the movie *Batman Begins*, clung to the cliff face like an ornate paper lantern in the sky. Throughout the week male competitors had been asking Zenia and I if we were going to race for first place. They seemed to be taking wagers on who was going to win. Surely, we wanted to know who was faster? Nope. Absolutely not. For Zenia and I none of this made sense. We had experienced the whole race together and would be finishing together. Even if this caused a headache for Stefan, who had to fashion another 1st place trophy from a miniature prayer wheel when Zenia and I crested that last ridge together, arms raised, sweaty and smiling.

By the closing ceremony at the Zhiwaling Hotel in Paro, saturated with Bhutanese song and dance, I realised I wasn't just ready to pack my bags – I was ready to move forward in life, buoyed by the friendships, the mountains and the knowledge that sometimes the gradual path brings the richest rewards.

As I chatted to the guest of honour, the former chief justice of Bhutan, debating the country's focus on national happiness, I reflected on my own life. Stage racing had helped me work out what I loved and what I needed to do. When things got too much, I had to to lose myself in nature and escape the city. At the finish line in Bhutan I had understood this, and that realisation had enabled me to move on. The race also closed an unfinished chapter for me – finishing a Global Limits stage race. The trauma of Cambodia was laid to rest and I knew I could safely race abroad again. With this closure I was able to move forward to the next stage in my life. I was ready to take a step back from travelling and adventure. The race's full title was Bhutan: The Last Secret and for me it was just that. My last chance – for the time being – to disappear and immerse myself in a meditative culture a world away from my own. I was finally ready for the change I had envisioned while contemplating my near-death experience in Cambodia. Career success was no longer my sole priority. Connection, family, nature – that's what was important to me. It was time to start our family.

Coda: Press reset

I emerged from my near-death experience in Cambodia hollowed out, my mind echoing with questions. I realised healing wasn't found in rest but in purposeful steps – so I resolved to press reset. Bhutan arrived like a whisper: prayer wheels, silent valleys and unexpected friendship taught me to move with purpose, breathing in each moment. I relearned my body's rhythms, trusted my heart's quiet yearnings and felt the weight of trauma lift with every shared smile. In the hush of ancient monasteries and beneath fluttering flags, I discovered that clarity comes not from racing forward, but from leaning into stillness. Bhutan didn't erase my past; it offered gentle closure, reminding me that renewal grows in connection – to nature, to others and to oneself. Emerging from those mountains I felt whole again, poised to embrace life's next phase with an open heart.

5

EMBRACE FAILURE

Spartathlon, Greece

'Avoid as much bullshit as you can. It will be flying around and they will be talking about 100-mile weeks, 150-mile races and as much macho crap as they can. What they won't mention is that none of them will have any idea about electrolytes, pacing and a number of other things. They'll be setting off too fast before panicking and fighting the cut-offs.' This was my baptism into the world of testosterone-fuelled hell. I'd inadvertently secured a place on the iconic Spartathlon ultramarathon, and my new coach was warning me what lay ahead. He couldn't have been more right.

I stared down at the dank grey bathroom floor. The hospital linoleum was smeared with a pool of water that appeared to have emanated from my body. Puzzled, I called the midwife asking if I still had amniotic fluid inside me. It seemed to be leaking from my undercarriage. 'No, Sophie,' she explained. 'You've just peed all over the bathroom. Don't worry.' Suddenly I understood what a pelvic floor was. And I no longer had one. Bursting into tears I felt mortified – and powerless. My son Donnacha was one day old and I was no longer in control of my own body. The shock was immediate. What if I couldn't run again? This was meant to be the happiest moment of my life – and it was – but it was undercut by a sense of dread.

For years, running had kept me sane and was the one consistent thing in my life throughout pregnancy. I'd run until I could run no more, only hanging up my running shoes at 30 weeks pregnant. But stopping was just temporary. I had every intention of lacing up those shoes as soon as I could, and now that hope had been ripped away from me. News from the hospital physiotherapist did nothing to allay my worst fears, and John swiftly ushered her out of the room when she nonchalantly suggested I might never run again. I was distraught by this news, and how she didn't understand why this was so important to me. It was another example of women being written off rather than supported to reach their full potential. But for now there was nothing I could do. And so, for three long months, I couldn't take a running step.

With no information available to support me, I was at a loss as to what to do next. Eventually, after weeks of googling, I stumbled across EVB (which stands for 'everybody') support shorts, which are designed to aid the pelvic floor and reduce bladder leakage. With them I could run without fear and gradually begin increasing my mileage. I only had one thing on my mind – I was determined to get back on the Ultra Trail du Mont Blanc (UTMB) start line.

I had originally applied for the 2014 race after pressing reset in Bhutan. I had heard about this iconic 171km challenge while in the throes of stage racing. It seemed to be a mystical beast of a race that stood at the pinnacle of the sport. It carved a path through the French, Italian and Swiss mountains, a place I longed to explore. It seemed the next logical step in my ultra-running journey, but I knew it would be tough to get into. Unlike my other races where I simply had to register and pay a fee, UTMB was incredibly competitive and securing a place was tricky. Throughout 2013 I had continued racing in order to acquire enough points to enter the UTMB ballot. At the same time I was trying to get pregnant and had no idea which life event would happen first. In my head I thought I'd get pregnant quickly, recover and have enough time to prepare for UTMB.

Unfortunately things didn't quite work out as I hoped. I became pregnant with Donnacha in early 2014, the same year I won a place in the UTMB ballot. Unable to defer my place, I would need to build up points to enter the ballot once more. The points worked in two-year cycles (though runners can apply every year), and to get a place in 2016 I needed to have accrued enough by December 2015. My previous points from 2012 and 2013 had expired, and I'd done limited racing in 2014 while I was pregnant. And so began the 2015 summer of racing in a bid to get two years' worth of points in a few months.

By six months postpartum I was relatively race fit, relying once more on my strong hiking skills to lower the impact on my pelvic floor. I wasn't aware of women's pelvic floor physios at the time and thought I just needed to resolve things myself. I had no coach, no training plan and no clue. The only structure I had was two strength sessions a week with my strength trainer, and I fitted in runs and spin classes whenever I could. I rocked up to races with a view to finishing them, rather than improving my performance. I was on a mission to accrue UTMB points and determined to march my way through as many races as possible. To qualify for the ballot, I had to run specific races and acquire 15 points in total. The number of points per race depended on the distance. With just one child to juggle, it was fairly straightforward. I'd sit in the car breast-feeding Donnacha before each race, while John went through the kit check on my behalf. A bemused volunteer often did a double take as John pulled a breast pump out of my pack while digging around for mandatory race items.

I ticked off Centurion North Downs Way 50 miler, Chiltern Challenge 50k and booked some annual leave to take a family beach holiday to Jersey to race 50 miles Round the Rock. I set off at 6 a.m. on one side of the island and finished on the beach outside the hotel, where Donnacha was playing in the sand in the late afternoon sun.

August brought with it the Ultra Trail Monte Rosa stage race where I covered 130km in three days in the snow-capped mountains of Switzerland before launching myself into a completely different climate, racing 275km (171 miles) in the desert at the Grand to Grand in Utah, USA. With barely any time to breathe, let alone recover, I was heading into October and the Autumn 100 miler through Oxfordshire and Berkshire. I was so laser-focused on gathering UTMB points I took barely any interest in my finish times. Completing the Autumn 100 in 22 hours and 41 minutes didn't mean anything at the time. It was 2015; I was still racing without a GPS watch and felt very much an amateur. In my mind I still wasn't a runner – I was a strong hiker at best – but that particular race proved to be a pivotal moment in my running career.

'You know you've run a qualifying time for Spartathlon?' my friend Krasse casually mentioned as we ran along the River Thames towpath. We had become great friends since meeting in Cambodia, and he'd patiently accompanied me on many stop-start runs during pregnancy when I'd constantly stopped for a wee. Krasse knew that even after all my frenetic points hunting and globe-trotting, I had been unlucky and missed out on the UTMB ballot again in 2016 – despite gathering enough points – and might now have to wait until 2018 to get an automatic entry (which occurs if you lose out on the ballot in two consecutive attempts). This was extremely frustrating, particularly after losing my 2014 place due to pregnancy.

Aware of the immense time and energy I had poured into securing a UTMB place, Krasse was attempting to distract me. Spartathlon? It hadn't even been on my radar. It was the race for the hardcore – those who ran 100-mile weeks, boasted about sub-three marathons and seemed surgically attached to their GPS watches. I was not one of them. I'd always seen myself as more of a hiker – good at going long and steady, but certainly not fast. Apparently, though, I had achieved a women's qualifying time at the Autumn 100, by completing a qualifying race in under 23 hours (the qualifier has subsequently changed to under 22 hours). And while that didn't guarantee an entry, it meant

I could enter the ballot. Even then, I wasn't sure I would get in. Or that I even wanted to.

The race stats were sobering. Only around 40 per cent of starters finished. Most runners – overwhelmingly male – were eliminated by tight cut-offs, the brutal midday heat or the sheer attrition of going beyond 24 hours. There was a particularly nasty cut-off at 172km, just after climbing a mountain. And that was 24.5 hours in for a runner like me. I'd never run longer than 24 hours before. But the prospect was tantalising. It was one of the most iconic and brutal ultramarathons in the world. Based on the legendary journey of the Greek messenger Pheidippides, who was sent from Athens to Sparta to request help in the battle against the Persians, the race retraces that 246km route. Runners leave Athens at sunrise and must reach the statue of King Leonidas in Sparta by sunset the following day, just 36 hours later. It's a race so steeped in history it feels almost sacred. You're not just running a course; you're stepping into a myth. The temptation was too strong. I entered the ballot.

The email pinged up on my phone. My palms were sweating at the mere sight of the word 'Spartathlon'. I took a deep breath and pressed open. *What???* The panic started to rise from the pit of my stomach, racing up my body to form an acid taste in my mouth. I had a place at Spartathlon! What on earth was I doing? The odds were entirely stacked against me. Within the Great Britain ballot (each country has an allotted number of places), I was one woman alongside 24 men. The whole race was only 15 per cent female. And I'd never run a road race this long before. My son was just one year old. I fell down the rabbit hole of comparison.

Blog posts boasted of men running 200-mile races, attending altitude training camps in the Alps and running very fast marathons. I couldn't compete with that. I was by now a mum of a toddler, working as CEO of a tech company, flying to Copenhagen every fortnight for meetings, squeezing runs into slivers of time between nursery drop-offs and client calls. Most of my miles came from running to work – Islington to Baker Street in London – before a quick shower and sitting down for the day. I'd often leave home at 4 a.m. to catch a flight and wouldn't be back until midnight. It wasn't exactly textbook training and yet, despite all this, I had the qualifying time. That meant I had earned my place. Still, this was the first race where I felt finishing was unlikely. What if I failed? But then again, what if I succeeded? What if there was a path to finishing? I decided to find out.

It was time to get serious and train smart. I needed a coach – someone to make every session count. That's when I turned to Robbie Britton, who'd met John during his recent Ice Ultra (John was predominantly a cyclist but loved stage races – particularly in cooler climates – so he did this one without me). Robbie was one of the UK's most experienced ultrarunners and had completed Spartathlon himself. He also happened to have a soft spot for the race. I sent him a message asking for help. He replied: 'You've sold yourself very short.' Doing his due diligence, Robbie had looked up my race history and pointed out that the longer the distance, the better I had performed, and I had been consistent. I hadn't really clocked that, but he was right. Robbie's coaching quota was full, but he couldn't resist supporting an athlete through one of his favourite races. He signed me up, but not before he sent me a warning about the macho bullshit surrounding the race.

The first step was working around my hectic schedule. We had just over five months and I had extremely limited time. It wasn't going to be about high mileage. We both knew that wasn't realistic. Instead, it would be about smart, purposeful training – focus over volume. Most weeks my training distance barely tipped over 50km, but I made up for it by filling my calendar with races. I was still using my trusty £5 Casio digital watch, refusing to become a slave to metrics. I could map read and follow markers, so I didn't see the need for a device telling me what to do. Runners around me always seemed to be stressed out when a checkpoint didn't correlate with their watch, while

I carried on breezily, assuming we would come across it in the next mile or so.

The turning point came when I nearly missed the last bus home after running the North Downs 50 as part of my Spartathlon training. I had promised I would be home for Donnacha's bedtime, but got chatting to another competitor along the course and missed a turn. Panicking as I realised the time, I hotfooted the last mile, grabbed my medal and legged it to the bus stop just as the bus pulled in. John gave me a stern talking to and bought me a smartwatch ahead of my next race. As well as being a great navigation tool, it symbolised something much deeper. I was ready to take my performance more seriously.

The South Downs Way 100 miler in June 2016 was a particular confidence boost. I ran it (wearing my shiny new watch) in 22 hours eight minutes, a much stronger effort than the previous year. I was still overtaking people at the end and felt like I could have kept going. Robbie was right. The longer the race, the stronger I got.

Then just as I was getting into the groove, a track session – my first ever – saw me goaded into running faster round a bend by one of the male members of my running club. He knew I had a Spartathlon place and it seemed like he was testing me – unfortunately I took the bait. I strained my hamstring and had to take nearly three weeks off. Robbie wasn't fazed. He told me not to worry about speed. I was never going to be fast – that wasn't my strength – but I had resilience and we'd work with that. During my recovery I missed out on a 100k race for training, but by this point it didn't matter – I had the endurance in the bag.

Three weeks before Sparta, I took part in the Médoc Marathon in France. It was not your typical pre-race sharpening event – unless your strategy includes drinking 30 (little) glasses of wine and dressing as Little Red Riding Hood. I ran in a velvet cloak, drank all the wine and danced my way to the finish line in just over six hours. Alongside me John – the Big Bad Wolf – joined in the running jubilations. Celebrating my first marathon with a pint of wine, oysters and steak felt like the perfect last hoorah before my big race. And although it wasn't part of the training plan – at least not officially – in hindsight it turned out to be useful stomach training. The night before the race, John and I attended the enormous pasta party and I made the most of the unlimited local wine. Being dehydrated and hungover on race morning forced me to adapt – a good rehearsal for running on a dodgy gut. I told myself it was heat adaptation too, as it had been a scorcher of a day and the velvet cloak was a heat suit in itself.

Race week arrived and I flew out to Athens alone. Robbie's toxic masculinity warning was ringing in my head as I headed to meet the team. We were all staying in one hotel, which felt like some supercharged macho all-inclusive holiday. It wasn't an official GB team but a contingent of British runners who had qualifying times and had made it through the ballot. Nonetheless they acted as an informal team, coming together before the race and posing in their matching t-shirts. Acutely aware that I was the only woman, I immediately felt like an outsider. The testosterone buzzed like static. No-one had heard of me – I'd never podiumed anything in the UK before – and I was told that the men had been discussing my race CV, concluding I was the least likely to finish. I'd been written off before I'd even started.

Meeting up with my crew – Krasse and Nick Kinsella, my strength trainer, whom I had been introduced to by my Marathon des Sables friend Ronnie – was a welcome relief. At least I had these men in my corner, even if they barely knew each other. Along with 400 other competitors we headed to race headquarters to get organised. Logistics for the race were unlike anything I'd experienced before. There were 75 checkpoints where you could leave a bag no bigger than a shoebox. We entered a vast hotel conference room populated with boxes numbered one to 75. I had decided to pack my race fuel in bright pink mail bags, knowing these would be easy to spot. None of the men at this race would be seen dead holding something pink. Opting for checkpoints ending with the number three (3, 13, 23 and so on), I deposited my series of snack-filled bags. Water would be freely available at the checkpoints so that was one less thing to worry about. There was nothing left to do but wait.

Chatting with the other GB runners before the race was a big mistake. They questioned my lack of training – I'd only averaged 60km a week for the last six months, including races, and my confidence rapidly started to dwindle. I felt like a sacrificial lamb brought to the feet of King Leonides. All I could think about was where I was going to fail on the race and how much I was going to let my crew down. I needed a pep talk. Calling Robbie, he once again told me to ignore the bullshit. 'You are absolutely in the right place. You deserve to be there. Run your own race.' Once again he was right. The numbers said it was possible. I just had to stick religiously to them. It was a series of checkpoints and all I had to do was stay ahead of the cut-offs. I could hike the mountains, run the flat and smash the downhills. Going off too fast would only lead to overheating. I just needed to stay an hour ahead of the cut-offs to give myself enough wriggle room if something went wrong. I had to keep my cool literally and metaphorically. Even with a 7 a.m. start temperatures would rapidly rise above 30 degrees.

Standing at the base of the Acropolis in pitch darkness, the air was filled with silent trepidation. Spotlights lit the columns above, casting long shadows across the narrow cobbled street as hundreds of runners gathered. I felt out of place and unconsciously moved to the back of the waiting throng. I was a short, muscular woman used to ambling along the trails and here I was surrounded by mostly tall, lean, road-running men. Sighing, I looked up at the ancient stones and thought of the weight of history. This was the same route the messenger Pheidippides had run. It felt sacred. I thought of Robbie's words: 'Run your own race. Don't let their bravado shake you. You're stronger than they think.' I repeated them like a mantra as we set off into the darkness. This was me against the clock. 'Trust the process. Keep eating. Keep drinking. I can do this,' I told myself.

The first few miles wove through silent streets past stinking oil refineries and chemical plants on the edge of Athens. The smell of oil and iron clung to the air. These toxic fumes were not the best start for my lungs, but I knew they would soon be behind me. My bright yellow waist belt was packed tight: water bottles, phone, familiar snacks and room for a head torch later. Others had tiny vests and barely any supplies. That wasn't me. I was there to finish, not gamble. As we edged out of Athens schoolchildren began to flood the route, high-fiving runners and asking for autographs. Everyone knew the significance of this race and as the city woke up it came out to greet us. Finally, at 24km, we veered left onto the coast road where the soft orange of dawn lit up the waves. The industrial bleakness gave way to shimmering beauty, the Aegean Saronic Gulf stretching wide beside us. I could feel my body relax. The cool breeze helped in the rising heat and I tucked into another small snack, checking off another box on my fuelling schedule. I was in control and on target for a 3:45 marathon. As the temperature soared into the 30s, I focused on dousing my head in cold water at each of the mini checkpoints. I couldn't afford to overheat. I ran on.

For the first 40km I had sporadic company, quickly chatting to other Brits as I passed them by. But most runners didn't speak English so just gave a solemn nod of solidarity before driving forward, head down. As time went by, the runners spread out, each choosing different checkpoints to restock their supplies. Despite being part of a wider team, this very much felt like a solo run.

Crossing a magnificent Corinthian aqueduct at 80km in, I couldn't help but marvel at the huge feat of engineering. I felt waves of vertigo and awe in equal measure. It seemed to rise from the earth like a monument to endurance. Clasping the handrails I guided myself across slowly, soaking in the significance. I didn't want to rush through this race like it was something to conquer. I wanted to feel – and see – every step. Easing off the bridge and around the corner, my crew met me with beaming smiles and an enticing Magnum ice cream. I had arrived at the checkpoint precisely on time – eight hours and 45 minutes. I was 45 minutes ahead of the cut-off and the timings eased off from here. Things were looking good.

Just 16km later I passed the Temple of Apollo in the heart of Ancient Corinth. Under the shadow of the tall Doric columns I reflected on one of the most revered Greek gods. Apollo has been recognised as the god of music, poetry and dance, and more significantly the god of divine distances, prophesying from afar. I hoped my own prophecy would be fulfilled – not with fire or fury, but with the soft, salt-stung kiss I'd plant on Leonidas' foot.

Hope burning in my heart, I turned right past the temple and the landscape changed once more. Neat rows of citrus orchards rolled out across the land, the scent of oranges thick in the air. I ran alone through tiny villages, relishing the calm before the climb. I knew the mountain was ahead. I wasn't afraid. I was looking forward to it. Hiking was my strength. This was where I held an advantage and could safely bank more time. The climb began with a long meandering road, covering 351m over 24km, heading towards ancient Nemea. By the time I reached Nemea, dusk was falling and I'd passed dozens of runners. I paused to dig out my head torch and gloves. The air temperature had dropped rapidly. It felt strange to be cold after baking in the sun, but I welcomed it. Cold kept me alert. I layered up quickly and pressed on.

At 150km, the village of Lyrkeia greeted me like a wild party. Visitors, supporters and crew were partying through the night – it felt like stepping into a Greek taverna mid-race. My name and photo flashed up on a huge screen to a roar of cheers. It was here that I devoured the best potatoes of my life. Slow cooked to perfection, the outsides were crispy and salty, the insides smooth and soft. Krasse sat me down offering up an array of more food. He'd set up a display of five different food groups, like a parent desperate to get their toddler to eat something. I picked at the sweets, crisps and fruit while Krasse refilled my waist bag, preparing me for the next stage. The mountain was calling.

With more than 145km in my legs and a full day under the sun, this is where the wheels might normally come off. The relentless 1000m climb from the base of Lyrkeia up to the majestic Mount Parthenion was a mammoth test of my resolve. It was 13km of up, up, up. Further and further into the darkness with only a headtorch to light the way. I'd been moving for 18 hours, my body was leaden with fatigue and yet I refused to yield to the mountain. I kicked into climbing mode, passing streams of runners as I hiked with purpose. My legs felt solid. I had climbing legs while most others only had road legs. The higher I climbed, the quieter it became. Head torches flickered like fireflies along the slope. I kept climbing, finding comfort in the effort. The top came slowly but surely. At the summit, I stopped. I was deep into the night around 3 a.m. and the stars glittered above me. The air was sharp and clean. I stood still, feeling the gravity of the place. This was where Pheidippides had met Pan, god of the wild. It was where myths lived. I raised my head to the sky and asked out loud for Pan's help: 'Please let me finish. I'm not done yet. I deserve this.' And with a final, 'Wish me luck!' I trotted off down the mountainside.

The descent was wild. Switchback after switchback on a wide track coated in gravel and loose stone. But this was my terrain. It was like dropping down Scafell Pike as a little girl. With child-like abandonment I let go, flying past Japanese and American roadrunners who made their way down cautiously. The sensation was liberating after the endless climb, and a warm beam of contentment filled me up from the inside out. I passed dozens of competitors. My shoes skidded, my legs pounded, but I was alive. By the bottom, I was grinning. I'd gone from surviving to thriving. I made up over an hour on the cut-offs and I still had more to give. Now only 80km separated me from King Leonidas.

By the time I reached the Plains of Tripolis at the 185km mark, everything felt surreal. It was the furthest I'd ever run continuously and a landmark moment, but all I could think about was moving forward. That vast, open stretch seemed to go on forever, exposed and unforgiving. It was early morning and I was still increasing time on the cut-offs, within touching distance of finishing under 33 hours. There was just one final climb to go and then I expected to be sailing through to the finish. Once more I power-hiked up the hill as other competitors insisted on running. I then passed them as they rested at the checkpoint and broke into a run on the descent. It was now mid-morning and the heat was becoming oppressive once more. But that was the least of my worries. The real problems were just beginning. I began hallucinating like crazy. The highway was punctuated with small white shrines, but my muddled brain thought they were the white t-shirts of the USA team. I kept trying to catch up with the American athlete ahead of me, thinking they were moving very slowly. I ran closer and suddenly the person evaporated, leaving behind a shrine. Together with the roar of trundling trucks I began to feel very uncomfortable.

Adding to my discomfort was the camber on the road. I was used to running on the canal path and, although it wasn't particularly smooth, it was at least fairly level. I had done very little road running, and moving for over 220km on the left-hand side of the highway meant my body had been constantly uneven. Suddenly I felt a tight constriction in my left quad. I had been shuffling along quite nicely, but, in an instant, I ground to a halt. There was no popping or sudden sharp pain, I simply couldn't run. It was like the muscle had turned to concrete. I was forced into a lopsided limp and if I tried to run the pain kicked in. Moving uphill felt OK, but flat or downhill was impossible. I was now hobbling in the blazing heat of the second day while a stream of runners passed me, sapping my confidence. They mumbled a few words of encouragement as the suffocating heat bounced off the concrete, but everyone was deep into their own personal battle, struggling onwards. This was my lonely pilgrimage to the bitter end. What I didn't realise until weeks later was that this was a deep-seated oedema. I had essentially developed a massive lump of fluid in the quad and there was nothing I could do but to keep walking. The oedema was so deep and so unusual that the sports medical consultant I saw subsequently used it to test his students. Question: How do you get an oedema deep inside the quad? Answer: Run on a camber for 200km. And so I walked. In pain. Grimacing. Limping. Struggling to put weight through my left leg. My crew were nearby but were essentially useless to me. They had no supports, no strapping, no tape. Nowadays, I always pack tape, but at the time I was completely exposed. There was nothing to hold me together except willpower.

I started doing maths in my head. Anything to stay focused. The distance markers were in kilometres, but I converted everything into miles and I estimated how fast I needed to go. All I had to do was limp at three miles per hour and not let the watch dip under 20-minute miles. An 18-minute mile was great; a 19-minute mile acceptable. But as soon as I saw a 20-minute mile pace flash up, I snapped to attention. Come on Sophie. Pick it up. My entire race had narrowed to this single, desperate metric. Ignore the pain. Don't worry about the injury. This was my A race. I had told myself at the start that I was willing to be injured for six to twelve months if it meant finishing Spartathlon. That isn't the case with every race, but this one was different. It was all or nothing. I was prepared to fail, but I would also do everything in my power not to.

Once I'd calculated the numbers I was in need of a new distraction. I began to sing. Not out loud – I couldn't risk wasting energy – but in my head. Before the race I'd tucked printed lyrics into mini zip-lock bags and stuffed them into my pack. We weren't allowed headphones for safety reasons, so these lyrics were my playlist. A personal jukebox of grit and determination. It was time to pull them out. *Eye of the Tiger* by Survivor, *Roar* by Katy Perry, *Strong* by Kelly Clarkson and even a little One Direction with *What Makes You Beautiful*. Those little bits of paper kept me going and I still find them today in old kit bags, crumpled and smudged from sweat. The internal ballads kept my mind elsewhere while the swelling in my quad continued to grow. All hope of a sub-33-hour finish was gone. But I still had time. I could still make it to the finish before the final 36-hour cut-off. With just 13 miles to go I put all my effort into concentrating on my watch, keeping my pace below 20. Those final miles were all downhill and naively I'd pictured myself flying through the last sections, legs churning, overtaking everyone in a triumphant blaze. Instead, I was hobbling. Every step was an effort. My quad screamed. Even the danger of being flattened by a lorry didn't register anymore. It was time to call John. I needed his voice to carry me through. He didn't say much – he didn't need to. Instead, he put Donnacha on the phone and my almost two-year-old sang *Twinkle Twinkle Little Star* to me. My eyes flooded. I felt every note ripple through me, peeling away the exhaustion, just for a second.

At the final checkpoint, where I could see my crew, I briefly stopped to prepare for the finale. For the first – and last – time in my life, I got finish-line ready. I changed my top, tied on a fresh headband and wiped the encrusted salt from my cheeks with a baby wipe. The salt had streaked through my tears like tiger stripes. I looked fierce and I felt raw.

But as I entered Sparta, everything changed. Crowds filled the balconies. Children on bikes tried to escort me in, wobbling as I moved so slowly they couldn't keep balance. 'Bravo! Bravo!' People were screaming from windows, leaning over railings, clapping from cafés. The air surged with energy. It lifted me. I wasn't flying, but I was floating. Wrapping a Union Jack flag around my shoulders I staggered towards the finish line. I might not have been selected as a GB athlete, but in that moment I felt deeply connected to my country and wanted to savour my only chance to represent it. Around me members of the GB team who had finished or fallen by the wayside cheered me on emphatically, as the tears clouded my vision. Wiping them away I saw him. The statue of Spartan warrior King Leonidas. My symbol of hope who had enabled me to stand firm against the invasion of doubters. Being a woman had not been a disadvantage. We excelled at these events. We prepared and completed them – but we were still poorly under-represented.

Crossing the threshold, I was immediately handed a chalice of water from the River Evrotas while an olive wreath was placed on my head. The spectacle was unlike any race I have experienced since. It was the perfect end to a 35-hour journey. And then – finally – I was invited to kiss the feet of Leonidas. The stone feet of history. Moments later I would be whisked away in a wheelchair and put on a drip. But in that moment, I was still standing. I had done it. And more than anything, I'd done it by ripping off the 'I am not a runner' label that had clung to me for years. The realisation sank in. I had been one all along. From the moment I signed up for the Marathon des Sables, through every race, every injury, every moment of self-doubt, I was a runner.

Just hours earlier, I had passed the Temple of Apollo in ancient Corinth, whispering a silent prayer to the god of divine distances. I'd asked for his blessing then. Now, with my fingers resting on Leonidas' foot, I smiled, knowing the answer had been yes.

Coda: Embrace failure

Spartathlon ignited something in me. It wasn't just a finish line, it was a transformation. For the first time I had allowed myself to embrace failure. I had stood at the edge of what I thought was possible – and then gone further. In doing so, I discovered not just what I could endure, but what I could become. It marked a shift from participation to performance as I explored what was possible with the support of my first coach. It was also an eye-opening experience of the male domination of extreme ultra-endurance. The lack of female participation was jaw dropping. There were so few running – most of the women I saw were either crew or spectators, waving on their male partners. Yet my story demonstrated just what women were capable of. We juggled families, full-time work and limited leisure time, and could still cross the line of a 246km race with tight cut-offs.

6

TAKE CONTROL

The road to UTMB

The Ultra Trail du Mont Blanc (UTMB) is more than just a race; it's a journey through the heart of the Alps, where the line between exhaustion and exhilaration blurs with every step. Spanning 171km across France, Switzerland and Italy, the course circles around the towering majesty of Mont Blanc, rising and falling over 10,000m. Walkers take up to two weeks to complete the same route along the Ultra Tour de Mont Blanc, pausing to rest in mountain refuges each night. But the UTMB is different – it's a relentless, non-stop test of endurance with a cut-off time of just 46.5 hours.

For years, conquering this legendary race had been one of my greatest running ambitions. In the world of ultrarunning, the UTMB race in Chamonix is the pinnacle competitive event – comparable to the Abbott World Marathon Majors, which include London, New York, Boston, Tokyo, Chicago, Berlin and now Sydney. Every year it is fiercely contested, with champions like Courtney Dauwalter and Kílian Jornet cementing their legendary status and securing lucrative sponsorship deals in the process. The course is notoriously challenging, with around a third of participants dropping out or failing to meet the strict time cut-offs. For me, it wasn't just about the experience, I was drawn to the challenge itself. Could I make it?

The first hurdle was getting into the race itself. The system works by runners accumulating enough points to be eligible to enter the lottery. In theory, this ensures those on the start line have the right physical and mental experience to take on such an extreme challenge. It also, more controversially, earns income for the UTMB itself, as other race organisers pay it to have points allocated to their races (the system has since changed, and runners now collect 'running stones' instead of points at UTMB World Series races; the more running stones you accumulate, the higher your chances of being selected via the lottery – and the more money UTMB earns). But even with the points accrued you are still fighting for a place. Entries are limited to 2300, and yet close to 9000 people now apply.

I first secured a spot in the 2014 race after diligently earning the required points at qualifying events and being lucky in the lottery. However, my race excitement was short-lived – I lost my place when I became pregnant with my first son Donnacha and UTMB organisers refused to grant a deferral. Turned down, with no possibility of appeal, I put my dream on hold. As I struggled to get back racing quickly enough after having Donnacha, I didn't have enough points and was only able to enter the ballot for the shorter 101km Courmayeur/Champex/Chamonix (CCC) race in 2015 which requires fewer points, but I failed on the ballot draw. Armed with a full set of points I entered the UTMB main ballots for 2016 and 2017, but I missed out again. All this time I was topping up my points at specific 100-mile races like the South Downs Way and the 126km Transgrancanaria Classic to ensure I met the race criteria. This was both expensive and time consuming, but I was determined to run UTMB.

The good news, of sorts, was that after two consecutive failed attempts to win a ballot place at UTMB, the race rules at the time granted me an automatic entry for the following year. When I missed out on the 2017 ballot yet again, I knew that 31 August 2018 would finally be my moment. After four years of waiting, I would stand on the start line I had been dreaming of.

Only it wasn't that simple. The spanner in the works was that we wanted a second baby. I'd been training hard for Spartathlon in September 2016, and we'd already decided to start trying as soon as the race was over. The first few months came and went with those painful single lines on the test sticks telling me that yet again we'd failed to conceive. By January 2017, I figured I'd soon get pregnant and have almost a year postpartum to train before hitting the UTMB start line in August 2018. Cycles came and went. Every time my period started I felt a sense of loss at what might have been. Long runs helped me switch off from the continual disappointment, and I was training hard for Lavaredo 120k, an ultramarathon in Cortina d'Ampezzo, Italy, circumventing the jagged Dolomite mountains. The spectacular race had recently been acquired by UTMB and folded into their World Series catalogue. It didn't require any points to enter, but it was a points qualifier for UTMB in Chamonix – my end goal. I was delighted as Lavaredo was also a bucket list event for me.

Then, weeks before the June race, I became pregnant. Somewhat ironically, given my experience with UTMB back in 2014, the organisers of Lavaredo were extremely supportive and refunded my race fee. John and I were thrilled I was pregnant, and the frustration of losing out on the race was quickly erased by the thrilling baby news. As a couple we had longed for a second child and now it was finally happening. We were not prepared for what came next.

I vividly remember the day we went for the first scan. We booked in early, so we could walk there on the way to work across London, and were nervously excited about seeing our baby for the first time. As I lay on the bed with cold jelly on my stomach, the sonographer moved the ultrasound monitor across my tummy. Something wasn't right. I turned my head to look at John and recognised confusion in his eyes. We both stared back at the screen. We were waiting for the rapid 'boom-boom-boom' echo we had experienced during our scans with Donnacha, but this familiar and comforting beat did not come. 'I'm sorry, but there's no heartbeat,' said the sonographer.

Anguish ricocheted through my body. I was devastated. We were devastated. Leaving the clinic in a state of shock I wiped my tears and tried to compose myself. John took me to Patisserie Valerie for a comforting pain au chocolat, but had to go straight back to the office after.

I didn't know how to process the news, so I did what I had always done and returned to work. No-one knew I was pregnant, so I suffered in silence. At this point I was the CEO of a tech company, and any hint of having another baby would have spooked investors and my team, despite my having managed it before. Grief would have to wait. We tried to carry on as normal, but a cloud loomed over me as I knew that any day the physical miscarriage would happen. A week later I suddenly woke at two in the morning in agony. It was happening. I desperately didn't want to wake John – I didn't want to make him relive his pain, so I crept downstairs to the bathroom. Muffling my screams, I figured there was nothing John could do to help. I just had to get through this, but the internal battle didn't stop there.

Soon after we travelled to Ireland to visit John's large family. We had been hoping to announce the pregnancy, and instead I found myself batting off questions about when I would give Donnacha a sibling, as if it was something I was holding back from John. I was dying inside, but tried to make light of the situation, brushing off the interrogation with comments about being busy at work. I couldn't tell them the truth – this was private to us and I didn't want it shared across Cork. And if the family knew we were trying for a baby they would be anticipating a pregnancy announcement every month, with messages of condolence each time it didn't happen. It was too much pressure to bear, but keeping the miscarriage secret was tearing me up inside and I needed to escape.

My idea of getting away from it all to allow myself time to grieve came in the form of a 105km mountain race. I was invited by my friend Matt Hearne to take part in Gran Trail Courmayeur, a race in the heart of the Alpine Aosta Valley in July. I'd met Matt swimming in the Serpentine while triathlon training, when John had clocked his MDS branded bag and struck up a conversation. We'd soon become good friends, sharing long runs and racing adventures across Europe together. The invite came at the perfect time. I just needed to run out my pain, frustration and deep internal sadness via a mountain adventure. I knew I could get round the course even if I wasn't at peak fitness, but I underestimated the technical terrain. Pelting down a hillside chatting away to Matt – about how I should probably stop talking and concentrate on the terrain – I stumbled and fell. My leg was covered in blood, but taking it in my stride I carried on, moving further into the wilderness. Soon after, Matt fell behind, unable to move as quickly as me in the heat which, like John, was always his nemesis. Pushing on I came to a remote part of the course, devoid of hikers, and I spotted a madness of marmots (yes, that is the collective noun). I stopped, enchanted by this one marmot, losing all sense of time. In that moment, staring at this strange furry creature, I felt a sense of release: everything was going to be OK, the sadness would pass and there was still so much joy in the world.

The next few miles became increasingly difficult and I felt unsafe on the loose, rocky ground. Aware that I had already taken a fall I was reluctant to put myself at further risk. By now it was dark and I didn't feel conditioned for the night ahead. While the plan was to complete the 105km race, the route passed via the 75km finish line. I rang John and consulted him on what to do. 'Did you get what you came for?' he asked. Yes. Yes I had. I had cleared my head, had time to myself and that was all I needed. Continuing in the dark, unable to view the magnificent scenery, seemed pointless. It was time to take control and stop. I timed out at 75km and made my way back to the hotel for a soothing shower. A few hours later Matt also returned, having made the same decision as me to time out at 75k. Keen to capture my marmot moment, the following day I dragged Matt around the local stores in search of a memento. I picked the cuddliest, squishiest marmot soft toy I could find and brought it back home to Donnacha.

While I don't have faith, something happened on those mountains as I stared into the eyes of that marmot. It was a turning point in my life: the moment I decided to take charge. With the UTMB place at the back of my mind we decided to embark on IVF. Medically, there was nothing 'wrong' with us. We had conceived Donnacha naturally – albeit after a year of trying and many months of Clomiphene, a drug which helps you ovulate more strongly – but I was now 35 years old and, as the consultant warned me, I wasn't getting any younger. IVF gave us the chance to take control and put the odds in our favour. To control the controllable. The stress of trying to get pregnant naturally and the subsequent miscarriage had ravaged my mental health. It was time to do something different.

An invasive period of drugs, injections, egg retrieval and general anaesthetic followed (the first time I had ever 'gone under'), which was a highly stressful time. But despite the poking and prodding, my analytical brain found the experience hugely positive. There were hormonal fluctuations and mood swings, but mostly I focused on the data: how many eggs were collected, how many were fertilised, what the ratio of eggs to a successful pregnancy were. Numbers were my wheelhouse and they helped me to follow the process and understand what was happening.

On our first cycle we were lucky to become pregnant and we had another son due in the middle of May 2018. The process had worked.

As soon as I saw those two positive blue lines I started calculating. Three months. My second child would be three months old at the end of August, the start of the UTMB. Being on the start line seemed inconceivable. Three months after Donnacha was born I was only just taking my first running steps, having had pelvic floor weakness after a difficult labour and assisted delivery. I had raced the North Downs Way 50-mile trail race when Donnacha was almost six months, stopping to express milk along the way, but three months was a completely different timeframe for recovery. And UTMB was an altogether different beast.

Despite the incredible excitement at finally being pregnant, my heart sank at the timing. It seemed that again I would miss out on what had long been a focus in my life – an experience I desperately wanted as a runner. But as John and I sat down to make plans for our next baby, he questioned my doubt. There was obviously a long list of reasons why I couldn't make the start line, but he wanted to discuss the reasons why I could. 'How can we?' he said. 'What would it take for it to happen? How can you prepare through your pregnancy to come out the other side as strong as possible? And how can we put plans in place that support you while our baby is young to get your fitness back?'

We debated at length. The answer seemed fairly extreme, but if the stars aligned there was a possibility we could make it happen. We split the planning into three parts. First, race-specific fitness during pregnancy – and preparing for an active labour. Second, getting my body strong after labour. And finally, logistics for the race itself. Despite the UTMB being, notionally, a running race, most finishers hike large portions of the course. Half, in fact, finish after the 40-hour mark, which equates to slightly less than three miles an hour, a fairly brisk walking pace on the flat. This is due to the race's technical nature. Much consists of rocky narrow paths continuously winding up and down the mountain, except for brief passages through small towns. With over 10,000m of climbing, even the fastest runners are reduced to hiking up some of the steep mountain trails, and less experienced runners have to pick their way slowly down the descents to avoid falling. The ability to run on the flat is less valuable in this race than the ability to hike quickly up a hill. Many runners who are forced to slow down and eventually time out of the race often struggle with their quads, the muscles at the front of the thigh above the knee. The constant impact from running downhill, known as eccentric loading, can leave their quads so fatigued that they are reduced to limping, unable to run or even hike at a decent pace.

Strengthening my quads to cope with this motion would be important in ensuring I didn't need to reduce my pace too much as the race progressed. In most mountain races, runners are permitted to use trekking poles. These enable your arms to help propel you up the hill, reducing the load on the legs. They can also be used to stabilise and reduce the impact on the downhill sections, which I knew would be important to keep my postpartum pelvis protected. With my strength trainer Nick I worked out a plan to meet these needs. It was the best we could do given there wasn't any pregnancy guidance on strength training. I had no female role models to turn to because I saw so few women getting back to strength and fitness straight after giving birth. To make my arms and back as strong as possible we focused on pull-ups, tricep dips on bars and full body movements using a weighted bar fixed at one end to the ground. For my quads we loaded a bar on my back and I lunged forward, pushing back to standing. Alongside these exercises we included kettlebell swings, tyre drags, single leg deadlifts, hamstring lunges and more to build strength and stability.

Over the months, some exercises needed adjustment. Eventually, my arms couldn't fit around my expanding belly for kettlebell swings, and I was less comfortable in squat positions. But for every muscle I needed to work, Nick found a way to do it that felt right. At eight months pregnant I was still training, doing full body pull-ups (these aren't recommended and I dropped them in my third pregnancy) and tricep dips on bars, while getting a whole load of funny looks from other gym goers.

Training during pregnancy was possibly the easiest part of our plan. I was working full-time, but with three-year-old Donnacha in nursery I could drop him off, powerwalk three miles to the gym and then get a strength session in before work. As CEO of the technology company I'd founded, with most of my team based in Copenhagen, I was lucky to be able to arrange my day like this. I'd catch up with the team by phone during my powerwalk, arrive at the office at 10 a.m. after a gym workout, work until 5 p.m. before pickup and then often work again from 8 p.m. to 11 p.m.

Having the goal of UTMB meant I prioritised my training sessions, making sure I was always focused on doing whatever I could to be ready for the start line. Even at nine months pregnant, I was walking quickly up the escalator at Angel tube station (the longest in London), using it as a quick hill session.

I decided early on that I wasn't going to run throughout my pregnancy. I had run to 7.5 months with Donnacha, and I figured running that late into my pregnancy might have been the reason for my pelvic floor weakness after he was born. In hindsight it was probably more the large episiotomy and the fact I had no idea what pelvic floor exercises were in pregnancy (or actually what a pelvic floor was). And the running I did when I was pregnant with him wasn't that much fun anyway – each run involved multiple laps of Victoria Park in London, passing the toilets each time. It was about 20 minutes' run from there back to my house, which I was always nervous about making in time. The weight of the uterus on the bladder makes you feel you need the loo much of the time during pregnancy, even if you don't. Knowing where the nearest toilet was always remained the priority.

So, at five months pregnant with my second child, I decided to stop running and to cross train for UTMB instead. I became a regular at my gym spin class, reserving the bike under the air conditioning unit as soon as the class opened, giving evil eyes to anyone who dared slip into the room before me and head in its direction. I set the treadmill at a high incline – up to 15 per cent – to walk quickly and did my interval training on the revolving stair mill. I found these exercises raised my heart rate very effectively without making me out of breath or incurring much impact on my body. By the time I went into labour – 10 days late – my body was strong, fit and ready for the biggest endurance event of my life.

Cormac was born in a birthing pool just as I planned, weighing 8lb 12oz. Like most second labours, it was a lot quicker than my first and, other than a few painful stitches by a midwife in training, a much better experience. It was too late to go home that evening, but my husband begged the nurses to let us out first thing in the morning. He rushed home to grab the buggy and I walked Cormac the 2.5 miles home, using the pushchair as a walking frame. I felt sore but I had control of my bodily functions, which, postpartum, was my first concern. It was straight back to training!

During pregnancy I had had a sense of control as I divided my time between work and training. This control was shattered as soon as Cormac arrived. Some parents find their babies have long stretches of sleep in the first few weeks, which allows at least some recovery to take place. We weren't that lucky. Cormac wanted constant feeding. For the first few days, even with John taking a week of his paternity leave, we struggled to get Donnacha, his older brother, to nursery before midday. The thought of getting to that start line in the Alps in three months' time seemed ridiculous given how little sleep I was getting and how little energy I had.

Work gave me little respite either. I had stepped down as CEO just before I gave birth. While I loved the role and my team, I realised the company was growing quickly and further investment needed to be raised. For me, being CEO at this stage was incompatible with being a present mother. I could do the job, as I had done after giving birth to Donnacha, but I realised how much family time I would have to sacrifice. I reflected on my learnings from Cambodia and what really mattered to me. The reason I co-founded the company was to develop technology that could protect children exposed to polluted air, and advocate for change to reduce pollution emissions. As the company grew, it became clear that making a positive difference was more important to me than making a fortune for investors that only focused on their monetary return. I agreed with the board to take a new role, as head of social impact and marketing, working flexibly while a new CEO was appointed.

The timing of Cormac's birth could not have been worse work-wise, though. Three weeks after he was born, I launched a partnership with Stella McCartney, shortly followed by our first consumer product (an appliance to clean the air inside vehicles) and then an installation cleaning the air in Marylebone train station in London. I recognised that these launches were a powerful opportunity to raise awareness about air pollution in the media, while also promoting the company. I didn't want to miss the chance to make a positive impact, nor did I want to let down our supportive partners, but I also didn't want to be absent from my baby and miss out on our bonding. I had to find a way of doing both. The only way to deliver these projects and get back to fitness was to have a lot of extra support.

In the first few weeks John took his paternity leave as a week off, then a few Fridays after that. We also engaged our previous nanny Margita, an incredible woman, who joined us when Cormac was just 10 days old. With Donnacha I had gone back to work when he was three months old, employing Margita's help at that stage. But this time around we needed her much sooner. She arrived at 7 a.m. each Monday and left at 7 a.m. each Friday, when Cormac and I had our solo day together. Margita was part of our plan and engaged enthusiastically, including making me healthy green smoothies to boost my energy every morning. John and I were able to sleep well four nights a week, which gave us enough energy for work and training. Margita went to sleep at 7 p.m., with me doing the 11 p.m. feed and settle, and then she brought Cormac to me in the middle of the night for a feed. The routine became like clockwork. I trained in the morning during a two-hour gap between feeds where I dropped Donnacha off at nursery, went to the gym and then back home to shower before Cormac needed his next feed. While I was pregnant we built a new home office, so once he was born I could work while Cormac slept and be on calls during feeds. I was working the equivalent of three days a week from when he was 10 days old, as well as training, exclusively breastfeeding and picking up my older son every day to spend time with him too.

I used to look at women in the public eye and wonder how they did it all. Now I realise. It is ruthless prioritisation and a huge amount of help. None of my UTMB prep would have worked without my nanny, Margita, and my salary, which paid her. My time was only spent working, training or with my family. Every

minute was optimised. Anything I could get help with I did –
extra hours from my cleaner Karley, my mum batch-cooking
for us, Margita running errands while Cormac napped in the
buggy. John stepped up too, focusing more on the boys, especially Donnacha, who suddenly found our attentions divided. It
was a rather extreme set-up, but without the support network it
would have been impossible.

Now that part one of the training was complete, I moved on
to the secondary stages. First, I needed to recover from childbirth and, second, I had to regain my fitness and strength to get
around the UTMB course. I was far more aware of my pelvic
floor this time around and religiously did my exercises during
pregnancy – which I continued every time I fed Cormac. Each
time he latched on was my cue to start squeezing. Then at six
weeks postpartum I saw a women's physio. She confirmed my
pelvic floor was still very weak, but said that – with the right
effort – I might be able to run in a 'few months'. In my head I did
the typical impatient-runner-returning-from-injury adjustment
and reduced that estimate to a few weeks. I already felt stronger
than last time. I restarted my stair mill training gently when
Cormac was 10 days old and after just a few weeks I could see
progress. During pregnancy I had been lifting not only myself
but my bump up the revolving stairs, and doing it without the
additional weight felt so much easier. Self-assured that I was
recovering well, I called my old running coach, Robbie, who
had trained me for Spartathlon.

I told him I planned to race UTMB in two months and asked
if he could help with a last-minute training programme. His
response? That I was completely crazy. He also felt unqualified
to support me. Having no training in postpartum fitness and not
having had a baby himself he – I now realise rightly – did not
feel comfortable giving me advice. Instead, he recommended
a mother of three and incredible ultrarunner, Edwina (Eddie)
Sutton, who was also an experienced running coach. Robbie
said Eddie would also say no, but at least she would be qualified
to say this. Robbie was right. Eddie initially tried to persuade

me that it was a bad idea, saying the injury risk was too high and there wasn't enough time for proper preparation, but the more we talked the more she realised how determined I was. Eddie decided that rather than saying no she would jump on board and help me get there in some sort of fighting shape. She knew I wouldn't take no for an answer and was excited to see if we could actually do it. There was no official postpartum return to running guidance at the time, so between us we agreed to set the main goal as getting to the start line and being able to run a few kilometres, with the second goal of reaching the half-way point in Courmayeur, Switzerland. We never talked about the idea of actually finishing the race, because that didn't seem possible.

Six weeks postpartum and I still couldn't take a running step without pelvic floor failure – otherwise known as peeing myself. My pelvis still felt like it had been pulled apart and any prolonged impact made it throb. Nevertheless, I was undeterred. I just wanted to experience the race, even if that meant only part of it. I was excited at the thought of spending time with my family in Chamonix, whatever happened. Living in Morzine, in the Alps, Eddie knew the course well and the training I needed for the terrain, especially the continual steep ups and downs. When I contacted her, I was already back weight-training with Nick, who had spent hours researching and selecting the best exercises to strengthen my core and undercarriage. Eddie added more dynamic exercises to these, as well as setting me tougher and tougher incline walking workouts on the treadmill.

I actually did very little running. Most of my training was strength and core work, plus exercise biking and uphill walking. At eight weeks I began to run a little, gently on soft mud-packed paths, once more wearing my specialist EVB pelvic support shorts. Little did I know that a game-changing device called a pessary would save my running career in the future. During the last three weeks before we left for Chamonix, I took the train to Box Hill in Surrey once a week. Box Hill wasn't exactly mountainous – the ascent climbed only 100m – but the aim was to complete 10 reps up and down via different routes without pain. This took about three hours each time. On the third visit I was trying to run downhill where it was less steep. This incurred much more impact on the body and my pelvis, with my pelvic floor needing to be strong enough to cope. I backed off when the throbbing started, walked a little, then tried again.

To leave Cormac for half a day for Box Hill training I pumped like crazy the day before to express enough milk for him when I was gone. My loop passed up via toilets and a café with a water stop, as staying hydrated, fuelled and not peeing myself was constant work. I then pumped behind a tree after my last rep before I took the train home, pumping on the return journey. He was still only having breast milk at this stage which helped me focus on getting the workout done so I could return to him quickly. Despite all my strength work I was still having pain in my pelvis running downhill. I knew I needed to be as gentle as possible on my body, but it was incredibly frustrating. I loved flying down the trails, arms flailing, mind racing ahead to choose the best line. I loved finding the point where I was only just in control, my legs cycling underneath me trying to keep up with my body. Having to walk down inclines supported by my poles would slow me down considerably and perhaps risk me failing to hit the time checks. But I knew I had to stick to the plan to get my body around in one piece. I had to stay cautious on the downhills and power up the inclines. I had it all under control.

One potential issue was the need to get a medical certificate signed, saying I was fit for the race. I signed up to a same day private doctor appointment on the last possible day to submit, hoping my postpartum bump would have deflated enough not to be noticeable. My vital stats were fine. He asked briefly about my training and signed the form. Phew. There were luckily no questions about whether I'd recently had a baby.

With Cormac approaching 15 weeks old we were ready to leave for Chamonix. I had achieved most of my goals. I was fit and strong but my pelvis was still sensitive over long periods of running.

Cormac was a happy and healthy baby, with Donnacha (now three) a proud, loving brother. The support I had around me, from my husband, parents, nanny, coach and friends meant I was in the best possible position to take on the UTMB. I had reached my goal. I had made it to the start line. I was mentally as well as physically healthy, having had the start line to focus on during pregnancy. But actually getting round the race? That would take a very different plan.

Coda: Take control

My journey to the UTMB was about more than just endurance – it was about taking back control. After years of setbacks, including losing my place due to pregnancy and repeated ballot failures, I refused to let circumstances dictate my path. When miscarriage and fertility struggles threatened my dream, I took charge, choosing IVF to regain control over my body and future. After my second son Cormac was born, I carefully planned my training, balancing motherhood, work and fitness with ruthless efficiency. I built a strong support system and adapted my workouts to strengthen my body postpartum. Every decision was intentional, from choosing the right coach to structuring my days around training and childcare. By the time I stood on the start line, I had already won in the most important way by proving to myself that, with determination and strategy, I could shape my own future on my own terms.

7

LEAN IN

Conquering UTMB and the Summer Spine

I sat on a hard bench in the packed square listening to nervous chatter spilling out in a dozen different languages. Hundreds of people kept filing in from all directions, marching down the cobblestone streets to squeeze into their starting position. Families milled around the edges, giving their loved ones a final lingering hug, before they disappeared into the maelstrom of polyester-clad runners. I looked down at Cormac, clinging to my breast as he sucked up his last supper from me. Little did he know that it would be 16 hours before he saw me again. And that it would be the moment that changed everything.

I had finally made it to Chamonix and was ready to take on the biggest race of my life, the UTMB. The A goal was to get through the first 10km, assess the situation, and then, if all was well, hike on to the halfway point. This was about experiencing the event I had dreamed of racing, only I was a participant now rather than a competitor. It was about seeing how far I could go, three months after giving birth, rather than completing the course in a particular time.

As always, race preparation centred around the kids. I wanted Donnacha to have a fun time rather than being dragged around to see me race. We rented a tiny old chalet with a garden – perfect for three-year-old Donnacha to chase around in. The days before the race were spent on family hikes in the hills, watching paragliders and breathing in the atmosphere. The streets of Chamonix were electric, with races of varying distances happening throughout the week. Each of the routes twisted through the French town, passing cafés and restaurants where thousands of spectators sat cheering. As we wandered through the streets, Donnacha was enthralled by the men running towards the finish line with their kids in tow. They were finishing the 148km Les Traces des Ducs de Savoie (TDS) race and savouring the final moments with their children. 'Mummy, that's going to be me!' shouted Donnacha excitedly, as he pointed to the families crossing the finish line. In that moment the enormity of what lay ahead sunk in.

I wanted my son to know he could do anything and that women were strong. I longed for Donnacha to have the same experience as all the other children crossing the finish line with their dads. We hadn't seen a single mum. My goal – the one I had discussed with Eddie over and over – had been to just get to Courmayeur, but at that moment I knew my only option was getting back to Chamonix. I needed to do absolutely everything in my power to run across that finish line with Donnacha. Three-year-olds don't understand DNFs.

The first hurdle was working out how to feed Cormac, who would only see me once in two days. He was still only having breastmilk, and although he would happily drink from a bottle, we had not tested him on anything other than my own milk. I worried about frozen milk spoiling on the journey, so we needed to find an alternative. Upon arrival in Chamonix three days before the race, we spent the first few hours searching the shops for a goat's milk formula, because we'd been advised that would be easier on his tummy when transitioning. Eventually John found goat's milk formula and Cormac wolfed it down on the first test feed. I then spent the next three days – between hikes – expressing as much breast milk as possible, so Cormac would have both options. Our part-time nanny Margita arrived the day of the race ready to care for Cormac, while the plan was that John would simultaneously look after Donnacha and drive around the Alps, ready to hand me a breast pump at various checkpoints. It was a logistical nightmare, but we were ready.

Many runners bemoan the 6 p.m. start time of the UTMB. It means you immediately go into your first night and have covered very little ground before sleep deprivation kicks in, but for me it was a blessing in disguise. The later start meant I could feed Cormac all day and give him a bedtime meal just before the race began. He was still feeding every three hours, but he could go for a longer six-hour stretch at night, which made things easier for John and Margita. It also meant I'd have less milk build up in the first few hours of the race. As the clocked ticked down to 6 p.m. I rose from the bench, giving him one last cuddle before handing him over to Margita.

Joining the back of the 2000-strong field I took a moment to breathe. I visualised the course and running towards the finish line with Donnacha. It was time to focus on myself, focus on my pace and stick to my plan. I set off at a gentle jog, trying not to feel frustrated that I wasn't further up the pack. Donnacha was waiting with John just on the outskirts of Chamonix and I stopped for a quick hug before I went off into the forest. All I had to do was stay ahead of the cut-offs – my final time or position were entirely irrelevant. This was a controlled hike and jog, aiming for under 44 hours to complete 171km. This meant I would be 150 minutes ahead of the 46.5 hour cut-off, which alleviated any stress that I would be timed out. My hiking felt strong on the inclines and for the first few hours I ducked into checkpoint toilets to hand express milk straight into the toilet bowl. Once the sun set, I was able to express under the cover of darkness straight on to the trail. By unhooking my pack, unzipping my jacket and hoiking up my bra over my swollen boobs I could release the pressure.

Before the race Eddie and I went over the key reasons I might fail or would have to pull out. If I didn't get rid of the built-up milk in time by squeezing it out my ducts could get blocked, leading to mastitis, a serious infection needing treatment. If I couldn't eat and drink enough to both fuel myself and keep my milk supply up, I'd be too slow for the cut-offs. But if I went too fast, especially on the downhills, the impact might injure my sensitive pelvis, preventing me from continuing, and meaning I would potentially have to endure a longer recovery.

The key was patience. Something I'm not particularly good at, but I knew in order to finish I had to follow the plan. I had no supporters on the course who could pass me my own preferred snacks at each aid station, and I couldn't possibly carry enough for the first 16 hours, so I needed to rely on aid station offerings. John was back at the chalet with the boys, and I hadn't wanted to ask friends for support because I didn't know how far round the course I would get. So, at each checkpoint I made myself stay until I'd eaten at least 300 calories, and stuffed another 300 calories of biscuits, cakes and crackers into a zip-lock sandwich bag for each hour I thought I'd be on the trail before the next station.

As the night wore on runners came hurtling past me on the descents, sometimes physically pushing me off the trail through their impatience to make up a few seconds. I stood firm and resisted the temptation to run, as well as the temptation to stick out a pole to teach them a lesson for their aggression. My pelvis felt extremely sensitive and I had to be cautious. Instead, I focused on what lay ahead, and looked forward to climbing Col de la Seigne and basking in the spectacular glacial views. I reached the peak at 7 a.m. and was met by a disappointing wall of mist. Nothing to see here.

By this point my breasts were feeling the strain of two missed feeds. They were throbbing intensely and expressing by hand was no longer making any difference. I had to get to Cormac. In agony I started the long descent into the Italian town of Courmayeur. For once it wasn't my pelvis causing the pain, it was my rock-solid breasts. Finally, after 16 hours away from my baby boy, I arrived at the checkpoint. I had reached the halfway point, but more importantly I could feed my son. And while my breasts were a mess, my legs felt OK and my pelvic floor felt manageable. Normally by then I'd be exhausted – depleted from the pace, but this time I'd taken everything slower. I wasn't racing. I was managing.

As soon as he spotted me John handed Cormac over the barrier, and I held him close. I could already feel the letdown in my breasts leaking through my bra. Making my way into the packed sports hall I couldn't see a single bench or table free. I snuck into a quieter cordoned off area reserved for some reason, but I reckoned no one would stop me when holding a baby. Cormac latched on giving me instant relief. My whole body exhaled. The ache in my chest eased, my heart rate calmed and I felt transformed into another person. I wasn't an ultrarunner grinding through the mountains. I was a mother, feeding my baby. And everything – even the race – took a backseat for a while.

It was during this moment of calm that Alexis Berg, the famous trail photographer, approached me. I knew how ridiculous it was, that I was there feeding my new baby, managing complex logistics because I hadn't been able to defer the race to the year after, when I would have fully recovered. I thought the photo might make UTMB realise what an unfair policy they had and that they would just change it straight away, but I certainly didn't expect it to go viral. At first, I looked up at the camera, in my usual smiling pose. Alexis clicked away and I went back to concentrating on Cormac. It was in that moment of connection, my eyes focusing on Cormac, that Alexis took his remarkable shot. Cormac lay slightly awkwardly across my splayed legs feeding from my left breast, while I expressed milk via a pump attached to my right breast. At my feet lay a giant yellow kit bag, the only thing separating me from the man with raised tattooed legs trying to sleep next to me. His yellow and black trail shoes matched his bag, bringing a splash of colour to the drab hall interior.

While the man napped next to me, I fed my son and John force-fed me an avocado sandwich. There was no time for me to sleep. My friend Matt – who had come with John – was in charge of my pack, taking out any wrappers, restocking it with fuel and changing the batteries in my headtorch for the night ahead. I had built time into my plan for rest and feeding, meaning I could afford to spend over an hour at the aid station. Usually, I would be in and out within 15 minutes tops, but I had a different perspective on time that day. Rather than worrying about wasting it, I savoured it, using the valuable minutes to their fullest to ensure both Cormac and I had everything we needed.

I'm not sure what time I'd have been aiming for fully fit – certainly under 36 hours, maybe much quicker – but being three months postpartum and full of milk put pay to any athletic goals. I was pacing for under 44 hours, two and half hours within the cut-off. This was at least eight hours slower than my pre pregnancy potential, but I didn't care. I hadn't come to race the clock. I came to finish, to stay healthy and to finally have my UTMB experience. Waiting outside was Donnacha, desperate to have a quick cuddle before I headed back off into the mountains. He wasn't allowed into the hall, so I made sure I had time to stop for a quick chat. Seeing his beaming, proud face gave me a power boost as I set off for the second half. I was determined to give him the finish line experience he wanted.

It was going to be a long, cold afternoon on the Italian Col Ferret pass. Despite the chill, the hours ticked by without incident as I navigated toward the Swiss lakeside town of Champex-Lac. That was, until midnight arrived and I'd been awake for 38 hours. Things then took a turn towards the bizarre. As I hiked through a dense pine forest, the trees covered in fluffy white blossom, my eyes began playing tricks. How lovely are the Swiss government? They've left duvets in the trees in case anyone needs to lie down and have a cosy sleep. It's just so kind of them! To my hallucinating mind the trees were draped with enticing duvets, a clear sign that my brain needed sleep. Still, oddly, I felt prepared for it. I'd been training for sleep deprivation for months – not intentionally, but by virtue of being a new mum. I was probably the most sleep-trained athlete on the start line.

Fortunately, John was my saviour once more, waiting for me in the Champex-Lac checkpoint with a breast pump and snacks. I subsequently discovered he'd had an absolute nightmare getting to the site in time, due to massive queues in the tunnels and the slow, twisty mountain roads. It was the early hours of the morning, but he'd driven all night to meet me. I was cold and struggling to discharge milk, but a lovely medic warmed me up with a blanket, which helped the milk to flow. I could barely keep my eyes open and the breast pump kept slipping out of my hand as my sleepy grip loosened. It was time for a snooze. After 20 luxurious minutes on a camp bed, John gently nudged me awake. I was groggy but refreshed enough to pump milk again and within a few minutes started to feel more alert. What struck me most about these aid station pumps was that no one batted an eyelid. Everyone had their heads down dealing with their own chaos – sorting gear, changing socks, taping up raw feet, stripping down, crying into their noodles. Bare breasts? People barely noticed. Some were half-naked themselves. I was surrounded by grown adults applying Vaseline to their chafed bits and desperately digging through their bags for salt tablets. Everyone was managing their own suffering.

Later, when the photo came out, some people asked why I didn't cover up. It was laughable. That's what breasts are for – feeding babies. And in the middle of a 171km race, when your body is broken and your baby needs milk, the last thing on your mind is modesty. I wasn't trying to make a statement; I was just trying to do what I needed to do. And honestly, if anyone was shocked, they've clearly never been to an aid station at 3 a.m.

As I left on the morning of the final day, I was filled with hope. There was only one climb left and I was in reasonable condition, all things considered. There was, however, a route change to contend with. A fatality in the mountains saw runners diverted along a technical descent over rugged tree roots. It made it much more treacherous – in fact, a helicopter was already evacuating someone who had a concussion after a nasty fall. This was not the dream finish I'd been hoping for. Instead of gliding down the mountain I was gingerly picking my feet up as I crossed root after root. It was painstaking work and my addled brain did not appreciate the challenge. Piles of people pushed past me, but I was determined to get down in one piece. I had mum duties to attend to and couldn't risk injury.

La Flégère was my final summit, and this time the weather was on my side. As I crested the mountain around noon the sun reflected off the crisp, hard-packed snow and I could see for miles across the Chamonix Valley. While eager runners threw themselves down the final descent, I stopped and sat down. Closing my eyes, I drew in the icy alpine air and held my breath. I was here. I had made it around the UTMB course with time to spare and I wasn't ready for the adventure to end. This was my moment and I wanted to hold on to it for as long as possible. I spent the next few minutes messaging Eddie, prolonging my time on the mountaintop, before setting off to rejoin my family. I knew that this was the end of my time to myself. At the bottom of the mountain I'd go back to being a mum again, dragged in multiple directions. Here I could just be Sophie, the runner.

Within an hour I was back on the edge of Chamonix looking out for Donnacha. There he stood, amongst the throngs of spectators, waving a silver and green windmill on a stick and wearing his tiny UTMB t-shirt. He'd looked longingly at those windmills in a store during the week and John must have given in to him while I was on course. Pulling away from John he latched on to my right hand, tugging me down the street. Slow down! Mummy is tired. Shuffling hand in hand through the bustling streets we were met with a roar of cheers and high fives. Donnacha was elated and lapping up every moment of the experience – just as I'd hoped. And then, from the corner of my eye, I spotted Cormac snuggled in a grey snow suit 100m from the finish line. Margita passed him across and I manoeuvred him into the crook of my left arm. Smothering Cormac in kisses, with Donnacha tightly gripping my hand, I shambled forward, oblivious to the noise and commotion around me. I barely noticed the people staring, aghast that a competitor was carrying such a small baby; that a mother had completed the course so soon after giving birth. All I could see was Donnacha's beaming face as he was swept up in the excitement of Mummy finishing a mountainous 171km race.

I crossed the line in 43:33:09 and was rewarded with an ill-fitting gilet. Now, where was that bench? As I sat feeding Cormac, a French midwife who was there supporting her partner wandered over, full of praise. 'You're just incredible. I've never seen anything like that before. I'm going to tell all the women in my clinic.' Up until then I hadn't really thought about the wider impact of my race. I hadn't even told anyone what I was doing. My parents thought we were just going for a holiday in the mountains and at that point I wasn't on social media. The reaction from the midwife made me realise it was probably something unusual, but it still didn't prepare me for what came next.

I didn't think much of the photo at the time. Cormac was three months old; I was halfway through the UTMB and just trying to do what I needed to do to achieve my goal. But a few days after returning home – having scoffed a box of deluxe French chocolates on the plane – Alexis got in touch. He was one of the best-known trail running photographers in the world, regularly capturing the likes of Kílian Jornet, one of the world's greatest ultrarunners, in spectacular locations. Alexis wanted to gather details, ask some questions and see if I was OK with the photo being shared. He attached a copy. I took a sharp intake of breath on seeing it. Brutally raw, beautiful; it represented the struggle I should not have had to have. The image captured me and Cormac lost in the moment during the height of the race. I noted he had cleverly framed us against a male runner fast asleep on the ground, legs in the air. That gave even more impact to what I was doing while the other competitors slept. I was overwhelmed with emotion. It was only a few days since I had crossed the finish line with both my sons – pulled across by Donnacha, with Cormac cradled in my arm – and achieved my dream of so many years.

Alexis asked me to share the story behind the photo with him. At first, I was not really sure there was a story. To me, I was just doing what I needed to do to finish the race and make sure my baby was fed. I was both a runner and a mother, and I was juggling, just as all mothers do. I didn't think I was doing anything particularly special. Finishing the UTMB was a struggle for all runners, from the first to the last and, that day, only two in three made it round the course. Like everyone else on that start line, I had my goal and as far as I was concerned, I had just done everything I needed to do to achieve it. What was strange about that? I only hoped that UTMB would change their inequitable pregnancy deferral policy on seeing it, so I responded – but I quickly forgot about it, immersed again in my busy life. What I didn't realise was the photo was quickly put out via the Associated Press (AP), a global news agency which publishers and broadcasters around the world subscribe to. This meant that any news organisation signed up to AP could run the image.

A couple of days later my phone pinged. It was my sister-in-law Jane asking me what I was doing with my boobs out on her Instagram feed. She'd had to do a double take and check the caption to confirm it really was me. 'What on earth were you doing running 171km up and down mountains when you've just had a baby?!' I'd forgotten we hadn't really told anyone we were going to Chamonix, never mind me running an ultramarathon while I was there. Since Cormac's arrival three months earlier, all our energy had been focused on him, Donnacha, my recovery and my work. Since Cambodia, I had tended not to tell my family what I was doing in advance to avoid them worrying.

I wasn't even sure what Instagram was. I'd opened an account a year before just to contact a local balloon company for Donnacha's birthday party, but had never thought to post anything. Once I managed to open it, I saw there were hundreds of thousands of people 'liking' my photo and tens of thousands commenting. It was already in social media and tens of languages all over the world – started by Strava and *Runner's World* magazine, who initially shared the story. I suddenly realised this was not about me running a mountain race that few have heard of. This was about motherhood and the struggle we have to juggle everything in our lives; the battle to keep our own dreams alive while doing the best we can for our babies. It wasn't about me at all – it was about the platform this image gave mothers to finally talk about their lives, to open up about the pressure on us and the difficulties we face.

Suddenly my inbox was full, with media requests from the UK, USA, Canada, India, France, Spain, Brazil. I took Cormac on a live interview on the BBC 2 *Victoria Derbyshire* show (where luckily he was an angel, despite my worries at him being sick on the posh sofa). I spoke at sports medicine conferences and my picture continued to be shared to millions of people. Topics such as breastfeeding, being a female athlete, the lack of support to get mothers back to fitness and more were suddenly in the spotlight like never before. To this day, that feeding station photo appears time and again in lists of iconic pictures that changed running and sport: The *Guardian* included it in a collection of 50 photos that reshaped sport; it was exhibited at the Saatchi gallery and the French Museum of Sport and it also became Strava's photo of the year.

Sadly, some of the coverage was less positive. *Runner's World US* ran an ill-advised poll on Twitter asking whether my breastfeeding during the race was 'gross,' 'a little selfish' or 'her business'. It was swiftly deleted after a barrage of complaints. *Slate* magazine called the poll 'dumb' and the backlash against this antiquated attitude was clear: women were tired of being judged for doing what men had done for decades – simultaneously being an athlete and a parent. There were cruel comments, as well. A small minority were disgusted and labelled me as self-centred for daring to leave my baby and go for a run. One headline in the *Daily Mail* announced Sophie Power 'shows no fear' – as if breastfeeding was something terrifying or embarrassing. In one interview a German journalist, a father of a newborn himself, asked me why I felt it was OK to breastfeed in public. He later apologised, explaining that his editor had instructed him to give me a hard time to find a new angle on the story. But the over-whelming response was support.

A particularly memorable moment was when I gave an inter-view to Anna Foster on Radio 5 Live. She asked me about the race and about the reaction to the photograph. I spoke about my hallucinations going into a second sleepless night, relieving my swollen breasts of excess milk behind trees and, finally, the over-whelming feeling of pride at crossing the finishing line with my two boys. Once the microphones were off, we had a very different conversation. We spoke of the struggle of being a working mum, of managing childcare and careers, of the mixed messages we are given by society, being told at the same time to 'lean in' at work, but also to create a perfect family life. We shared our tips, tricks and shortcuts – how we both managed it all, how we both tried to find that elusive balance in our lives. And suddenly we realised that surely *that* should have been the interview our listeners heard.

This was reflected back at me via thousands of messages that came in from women who saw themselves in the UTMB image. Some told me they'd felt they had to choose between motherhood and themselves. Men contacted me too, asking how they could become better allies to their female partners. Race directors reached out, asking how they could improve their policies for women and telling me that they were hastily writing pregnancy deferral policies, having never thought about them before. One photo had sparked a world of change. I hadn't intended to become a symbol. I'd just wanted to do the event. I had trained hard for that start line, despite knowing I wouldn't be racing it. My goal was to see how far I could go and to feed my baby. But suddenly my actions were starting global conversa-tions on maternal identity, female endurance and what women's bodies are capable of. I found myself asked to speak on panels, in interviews, on podcasts. People were paying attention. Not just to me – to the wider issue. The image had cracked something open. And for me, it wasn't just a fleeting viral moment. It might have been 15 minutes of fame, but it was also the awakening of something that changed my life.

Suddenly Jasmin Paris was contacting me asking for advice on expressing milk before she competed in the Spine Race. I told her that staying hydrated and warm were the most important things because, as I found out in Champex-Lac, it was very hard to get breastmilk flowing without these. Jasmin went on to win the race outright and smash the course record. Her amazing story also quite rightly garnered worldwide coverage, as the media finally started to take notice of women's sporting achievements. Meanwhile, my family and I were invited to the women's half-marathon in Madrid, where I was awarded an inspirational mother award by the mayor. More stories appeared in the press about women returning to sport stronger following pregnancy. The culmination of these events uplifted me. It felt like a shift was happening, led by a movement of mothers.

The seed of SheRACES, a conduit to make sport more inclusive for women, had been planted – I just didn't know it yet. I was not comfortable with the attention – we were a private family – but felt I had been given an opportunity to help others and I needed to lean into it. This was my chance to give a voice to mothers, speak out on injustice and simultaneously show the strength of women while highlighting the barriers they face. What began as a pushback against the lack of pregnancy deferral policies rapidly became about so much more. It was about recognising the physical capabilities of women, while acknowledging our differences. It was about removing barriers and elevating female athletes. It was about creating fairness and opportunity for women in sport. I was filled with an overwhelming feeling that I wanted to ensure I did everything I could with my newfound platform. It had to mean something. I had to make a difference.

At the same time, I was being pulled in so many different directions. I was working almost full-time, the kids were still tiny and now my head was swimming with ideas. My goal had been to tackle air pollution in London for the sake of children's lungs, but we were in the process of moving out of the city to a more child-friendly environment in Surrey. The daily threat of air pollution was not always top of my mind. Suddenly my eyes had been opened to a new world of advocacy, one which could impact women on a global scale. During an interview with a leadership organisation I was looking to join, the interviewer commented that he felt my heart was more in women's sport. This took me by surprise, because my head had been so laser-focused on air pollution. But in my heart, I knew they were right. Things were starting to tilt in a new direction.

This change in perspective was heightened during a bizarre encounter at a charity talk a few weeks after UTMB. I found myself speaking alongside pro runner Tom Evans, at the time sponsored by Adidas and Red Bull, at an Impact Marathon event. Impact Marathons are incredible races that raise funds for high impact local projects, alongside epic race experiences in countries from Guatemala to Nepal. Nick Kershaw, the founder, is a close friend and invited me to share my UTMB story as part of the evening.

There was Tom, who had just won the 100km UTMB Courmayeur/Champex/Chamonix (CCC) race, talking about his strict nutrition regime. Once a fortnight he would treat himself to an almond croissant. One croissant. A fortnight. He optimised absolutely everything in his life to ensure he came out on top. And there I was, a mum of two who had come in only a couple of hours ahead of the UTMB cut-off, 99th woman. My strategic pre-race nutrition plan had been stuffing my face with Nutella on toast several times a day. It was laughable. There was no way as a working mum that I could ever have his kind of commitment. But at the back of my brain a thought was itching away. What if I could be a bit more 'Tom' in my approach? It was an intriguing thought. Inspired by his dedication in my head I developed the 'Tom Evans spectrum', something we have subsequently chuckled about together as our paths have recrossed. If a Tom Evans performance was 100 per cent on the spectrum, where did my efforts fall in comparison? Just finishing an event would sit around 50 per cent, but what would 60, 70 or even 80 per cent look like? Could I ever reach 80 per cent? And what would I need to sacrifice? I'd really have to dial down other aspects of my life and reconsider my priorities. Something would have to give. But maybe it could. And if so, what could I achieve as a runner?

For 18 months I'd been riding the wave of UTMB. There had been a huge build-up throughout pregnancy and into postpartum training, which had only swelled further once the unexpected media storm hit. For years I'd dreamed of completing the challenge and, rather than the usual post-race blues spent seeking a new adventure to sign up to, I'd extended the high through months of talking about it. My career had also taken an about-turn. I'd quit my marketing post in the tech firm, moved out of London to Surrey and begun freelance consultancy work. I was doing ad hoc advisory work off the back of UTMB and was constantly thinking about my future. Things had been hectic but, as always, I needed a fresh goal to keep me motivated to run. When Cormac started weaning I knew things would be simpler and I could throw myself into something new. I briefly considered a Bob Graham Round – a fell running challenge in my second home of the Lake District. It covers 42 of the highest peaks around a 106km circuit with a total ascent of 8200m. Most participants attempt to complete it within 24 hours, but once again the logistics would be tricky. I'd need to go away to recce the route, and the attempt itself would rely on family and friends crewing and pacing me. I really didn't want the mental planning load so soon after UTMB. I needed a self-sufficient adventure where I could just turn up on my own and run.

The Montane Summer Spine Race, along the Pennine Way and scheduled for June 2019, had huge appeal. I had never run for more than 48 hours continuously or attempted anything longer than 160km. The Spine was 431km with a seven-day window. And it seemed far more sensible than the more iconic

Winter Spine Race. I knew from Iceland that the cold did not agree with me. (I've previously mentioned I have Raynaud's disease, which affects blood flow to my fingers and toes, and gives me a higher-than-average hypothermia risk.) Training would also be fairly straightforward, as we'd recently moved to Surrey and I could work on my hiking speed in the surrounding North Downs. With 10,000m of elevation I surmised that it was more of a hiking than a running race, which lent itself to my strengths. Using my newly formulated Tom Evans spectrum I decided that this was about experiencing and getting round the race, rather than performance goals. I wanted to do the race, but it wasn't going to take priority over my life. It sat quite comfortably at around 50 per cent on the scale as I calculated my pace around childcare. There was no way John could take the week off work, but my parents had agreed to help with the kids. However, there was a limit on how long they wanted to stay for. That meant I had to complete the Spine in five days. Once more my race strategy was designed around childcare needs ahead of anything else.

Having tackled UTMB three months postpartum, I expected the Spine to be relatively straightforward, even if the checkpoints were 40 to 50 miles apart. I was completing it in the summer, after all, and was well prepared for hiking steep gradients. In hindsight, I was incredibly naïve and ill-prepared. What I hadn't anticipated were the bogs. Summer bogs. Twenty-four hours in, my feet were completely shredded and felt like they had doubled in size due to constantly being submerged in water (I had no waterproof socks). Fortunately, for the first 48 hours I was distracted by the company of Estonian philosopher Paertel Piirimae. Having studied philosophy in my first year at university, I had forgotten most of it and took the opportunity to ask for a refresher in Descartes and Milne. Wondering whether the tree has fallen in the forest if you can't see it while hallucinating is one of my stranger ultra memories.

In a neat cycle of comparison Paertal had finished UTMB the same year as me, some five hours ahead of my time. At the Spine I pulled away on day three, finishing four hours before him. But while I journeyed with him, I was enormously grateful for his company – and never more so than on day two as we climbed Cauldron Snout. The rocky path rose above an engorged river, overflowing with flood water. One slip on the treacherous rock face and I'd be washed away by the extreme current. I was petrified and wondered what on earth I was doing. Had I been there on my own I would've had to wait hours for the next racer to come along to help guide me up the steep climb. There was no way I would have attempted it on my own. Fortunately, Paertal and I were able to navigate it together, working out the safest steps to take where the path had most traction.

On days three to five, when I did end up running long stretches on my own, the only debilitating obstacles were the stiles. These were stone steps protruding from the walls leading up to a tiny gap at the top. My heavy feet had swollen so much that squeezing my massive size 8.5 Hoka shoes (I'm usually a 7) through the hole was a huge undertaking. They constantly got caught in the gap, making me wince and exhale a line of expletives. The whole painful manoeuvre took an inordinate amount of time. Hiking and running wasn't much better as my feet were so filled with fluid that it felt like I was moving on stumps laid on a bed of needles. Every now and then I'd stop in a field and focus on a deep breathing technique to manage the pain. I'd been invited on a *Slate* podcast the week before where 'Iceman' Wim Hof had taught me to manage pain during the upcoming race. While I ignored his cold-shower preparation advice, I made sure to remember his recommendation to breathe in through the nose for two, huff out all the air through the mouth and repeat 20 times.

I had few moments of respite on the course. Stopping to rest and elevate my poor feet wasn't an option. In other races I would have had two more days to finish, but this time I had a deadline to meet – grandparents in Surrey who needed to be relieved from childcaring duties – and this was the motivation to keep moving, despite my severe discomfort. However, this tactic would only take me so far. Like in UTMB the year before the sleep demons were coming to get me. After wolfing down a tray of the legendary Spine lasagne, I did manage to grab three hours' sleep at the bunkhouse in Alston, 290km into the race – until the delicious smell of buttery toast wafting through the cabin woke me from that deep slumber. I was starving again, and happy to relieve race staff of two large plates of toast while my feet were attended to. A medic covered my feet in a fluffy webbing I'd never seen before – but it worked a treat. I had heard that the care and consideration of volunteers on the Spine was unlike any other race – and together with the kindness of strangers along the route – it surpassed my expectations. A particular highlight was a local triathlon club which took bacon sandwich orders at the bottom of a hill. These were then radioed to the summit, and a team of hardy volunteers with a camping stove were ready with my sarnie and cup of tea by the time I arrived at the peak. That kindness and sense of community was remarkable.

As I left the Alston checkpoint I was struck by the cold. I had never expected to be this close to hypothermia on a summer race. I had to keep moving; I couldn't get too cold. On Cross Fell, the highest and most exposed part of the course, the mist came in and I could see absolutely nothing. I could barely see two metres in front me, and had to rely on the GPS tracker on my watch for navigation. Fortunately, the days of the Casio watch were long gone. Despite the awful conditions, I still felt an immense sense of adventure and the simplicity of being out in the wilds on my own, without having to worry about rushing to the next stop to breastfeed my baby. It was exactly the reset I needed after UTMB.

I finally reached the never-ending Cheviots climb knowing I had less than 20 miles to go. Running under a full moon I sensed an eerie presence nearby. Suddenly the shadowy figure of a man appeared from nowhere and started running towards me. For a second I froze on the spot, absolutely terrified. I had no sense of what was happening or who he was. The figure kept moving towards me, lifting something in the air. The object glimmered in the moonlight. Is that a…camera? The tension in my body dissipated. It was the race videographer, not an axe murderer. Relieved to see a friendly face I allowed him to film me and mumbled a few incoherent words about how I was feeling.

Leaving behind the first person I'd seen in hours was hard, especially since it was now 3 a.m. in the morning. To keep my mind occupied I listened to the soothing tones of Michelle Obama reading her audiobook. As I hopped along a series of stone slabs I was drawn to their smooth faces. They looked like lovely pillows. Lying down, my head on the cold bedrock, I slipped into a short nap. I'd been desperate to continue, but just couldn't stay awake any longer. Revived by a few minutes face-down on the slabs, I stumbled up and lurched forward onward to the next checkpoint. I arrived at the hut just as the sun rose, bringing with it a glorious pinky-orange glow that lit up the valley with celestial grace. A cup of tea in hand I sat on the wall admiring the stunning view. This is what I came for. But I couldn't linger too long – I had a race to finish and a train to catch.

Power-hiking the final stretch I was approached by the videographer again. 'Can you run down the final bit?' he asked. I scoffed. I could barely walk let alone run. All my weight was pushed on to my poles in a fruitless bid to take the strain off my feet, which by now were excruciatingly painful. Hobbling across the finish in 119 hours and 6 minutes, I was immensely relieved. This time around the challenge had been all mental – rather than physical. But still I had managed to achieve my main goal of making it round in time to catch my specific train home. I even had enough spare time to have a shower, and therefore spare my fellow passengers my stench on the train home. There was also the added bonus of coming second female, behind the formidable Sabrina Verjee, who had won the race outright, 30 hours ahead of me.

This was the longest non-stop race I'd completed, and pacing-wise it had gone to plan. Normally I would forgo a race t-shirt, opting to plant a tree instead, but this time I was excited for it. I had earned it. My race had been timed to perfection and I'd slogged through days of painful feet. I couldn't wait to wear my t-shirt with pride. That piece of clothing was a massive deal, but it didn't fit. It was a male size small – and was enormous on me. Totally unwearable. I burst into tears the moment I put it on. I'd recovered from having a baby, trained extremely hard, suffered for days on the course and the least I deserved was a t-shirt that fitted me. Why was it so hard? It felt like every race I entered was only designed for men. A man could defer a race place due to injury, but a woman couldn't if she was pregnant. A man could have a t-shirt that was the correct size for his sex, but a woman couldn't. And women were being physically pushed off trails to make space for men. Something needed to change.

Coda: Lean in

At UTMB I chose to lean in. Three months after giving birth, I wasn't racing for time or trying to prove anything. I was there to experience it fully, to show up as both an athlete and a mother. Feeding Cormac at Courmayeur, letting Alexis take that photo, I didn't shy away from what that moment represented. I allowed it. I lingered on the final hill, not rushing to the finish, but pausing to take it all in. The mountains, the journey, the meaning – I could have kept my head down and pushed through to the finish, but I didn't. I leaned into the emotion, the spectacular views, the achievement. And that photo? It became something bigger. It wasn't just about me any more – it was a catalyst. I used the moment to call out inequality, to start conversations and to push for change. I leaned in and everything shifted.

8

BE FLEXIBLE

An active pregnancy

I was still running the day my waters broke. As the crisp November sun shone through my upstairs gym window, I raised the incline to 10 per cent and began to hike. My body was trying to tell me something. I was almost 39 weeks pregnant, and after a mile of jogging my body finally said, 'No more running'. Walking the rest of the session up the gradual incline, I watched my feet move satisfyingly step after step. I had grown accustomed to the hypnotic whirr of the treadmill since my last outdoor run three weeks ago. We were entering another 2020 lockdown, and though I preferred the rush of fresh air when running out on the trails, the treadmill felt less impactful on my body. It also made my regular bathroom stops far easier – no more searching around for bump-sized bushes. In the comfort of my own home I could manage five gentle miles, stopping to walk or go to the toilet every so often, with no risk I'd find myself stranded if I couldn't go on.

Compared to my previous two pregnancies, carrying Saoirse had been an athlete's dream. I expected my body to reject running at six months and had actively planned alternative exercises, but most days I was still feeling great. I'd regularly run six miles after school and nursery drop-offs (Donnacha was now five, and Cormac two), and I was still lifting weights and training on the bike. Learning the hard way from my previous two pregnancies, I was determined to train and recover properly for my third. I had always listened to my body and never put my baby under stress, but some of my training had not been adapted for pregnancy. Doing pull-ups at eight months pregnant with Cormac seemed impressive to me at the time. However, in hindsight it wasn't my finest hour as I didn't make any modifications to prevent my abdomen from doming. It was about finding the line — and not crossing it.

I was also aware that this time my training would be far more public, potentially a source of intense interest for journalists and social media alike, as I was determined to share the ins and outs — a case study of one — so other women could learn from it. I started blogging and posting photos of my pregnancy journey, being brutally honest about the highs and lows of training. I knew exercise was incredibly important for the health of my baby — and me. Countless studies had shown mother and baby's health improved when pregnant women exercised, and it was far worse to sit idly at home (unless you had a medical complication). Research had also debunked the unfounded myth that vigorous exercise was dangerous for pregnant women and their unborn babies. High-intensity interval training had actually been found to improve umbilical blood flow and promote sleep in pregnant women without any adverse effects. Armed with this knowledge, I knew staying active during pregnancy was non-negotiable. But it wasn't always easy.

During my first pregnancy with Donnacha, I'd had to stop running at seven months as my aching body had had enough. The frustration continued postpartum as I suffered from pelvic floor issues leading to embarrassing leakage. Running was off the cards for three months until I discovered pelvic support shorts. I had similar problems with Cormac, three years later. Running was halted prematurely at five months pregnant, because of pelvic pain, so I ramped up the hiking and weight training in preparation for my infamous UTMB attempt. This time it would be different.

Since my UTMB photo I'd met some of the world's leading experts as part of my role as ambassador for the Active Pregnancy Foundation. I wanted the best professional guidance available – no more making it up as I went along – and what better person than the woman who had co-written the guidance on returning to running postpartum, pelvic health physio Emma Brockwell? Alongside my terrific coach Eddie Sutton, the duo became my two-headed Jiminy Cricket, whispering in my ear when I was tempted to push too hard. The three of us collaborated, chatting through training plans and goals, which not only helped to build my confidence, but also gave me boundaries. I listened to them, took their advice seriously and felt this pregnancy would be different. Emma had my back and I assumed everything would slot into place.

I even convinced running brand Hoka to make a film about my experience, entitled *The Journey from Pregnancy to Performance*. The idea was that it would chart my fitness journey through pregnancy, birth and postpartum to give a positive but realistic portrayal of active pregnancy. The film grew out of my desire to see more images of women being active while pregnant. Working with the Active Pregnancy Foundation – a science-led charity that aimed to remove barriers to activity – made me realise how rarely I saw photographs of pregnant women exercising. I felt strongly that these images needed to be available to normalise active pregnancy. Pregnant women were afraid of exercising because they rarely saw others doing it – and yet it was vitally important for the health of their baby and themselves.

Hoka had made a short film with me after my infamous UTMB race, showing me getting back to running following the birth of Cormac, and I initially approached them asking if they would sponsor some photos of me running while heavily pregnant. One golden morning, local photographer Phil Hill took a series of pictures of me running against an idyllic sunrise. The photos were incredible, but they weren't enough. We needed to show the whole journey including postpartum recovery, so Hoka bravely agreed to fund the film, not knowing what the outcome would be. Everything seemed to be falling into place. I had expertise on my side, I was making a groundbreaking film and I assumed I'd be racing 50km within 12 weeks of giving birth. After all, I'd done the 170km UTMB when Cormac was just three months. What could possibly go wrong?

My first goal was just to have a happy and healthy pregnancy, staying as active as possible, as much for my mental as my physical health. I'd found out I was pregnant just days before the first 2020 lockdown, and we moved house two weeks later. Our lives were in boxes, I was juggling homeschooling a five-year-old, keeping an 18-month-old entertained and trying not to throw up everywhere. My training plan kept me sane, the one part of structure in my week. Having that plan gave me permission to prioritise myself for short periods of time each day, a mental lifesaver in the groundhog days of lockdown. With gyms now closed, John bought me a treadmill as a pregnancy present. One of the bedrooms in our new home had previously been set up as a gym, and we threw in all the bits of random weights and equipment we'd accumulated over the years, counting our blessings that we were still able to exercise while confined indoors. When Cormac napped, I could have him on the monitor with Donnacha playing in the gym with me. With the world outside in chaos, with my homelife in chaos, at least my pregnancy was going according to plan. I had the perfect home set-up, expert support around me and no medical contraindications to exercise. The problem was I'd forgotten that pregnancy rarely all goes smoothly.

This realisation hit me in the form of a urinary wave. I was 15 weeks pregnant and halfway into a two-hour-long run along the sandy tracks of the forested North Downs Way. Suddenly my pelvic floor felt like it had completely disappeared. Anxiously I dove into the bushes for yet another wild wee. I felt completely out of control, ashamed and helpless. I wasn't an 80-year-old woman, so why couldn't I control my bladder?! I felt like I had failed. I had definitely been slacking on my pelvic floor exercises, but didn't expect it to fall apart like this. Was running over already? I had months to go. It couldn't be over yet! All I could do was continually stop to wee in a feeble attempt to prevent my pants filling with urine. I cried all the way home.

Doubling down on pelvic floor exercises, I put my long run into a mental box of things to forget and focused on the next block of training. I can do this. I've done it before. I am strong. But my reprieve was short lived. Just a week later I was walking the kids home from school down a steep grassy hill. Suddenly it hit me. A wave of sharp pain jolted through my pelvis. Physically stopped in my tracks, I stood helplessly trying to focus on deep breaths. Tentatively, I stepped forward a few metres, trying to catch up with the boys. The pain attacked again. Taking another big breath, I focused on getting to our front door. It was only a minute away and, somehow, I managed to stumble back, the boys eyeing me with concern the whole way.

Reaching home, I sent the kids to their playroom. I needed to get rid of the pain. Lowering myself on to the living room rug, I stretched out into the yoga position Child's Pose. Slowly the pain subsided, dissipating from my pelvis in flutters of discomfort. After 30 minutes of lying on the floor I was able to move again. Fortunately, the incident appeared to be isolated, but I took it as an unmistakable warning – my body was urging me to ease the pressure on my pelvis. I needed to be flexible and adapt according to my body. Digging out my pregnancy pillow and waist belt, I vowed to support my bump even when sitting or lying – which, as a busy mum, was hard to implement. But with my pillow companion, the next few weeks rolled by smoothly, steadily rebuilding my confidence.

The rollercoaster journey continued. At 18 weeks I was feeling invincible again and in need of a challenge. The waist belt was supporting my bump extremely well and I never went out of the house without it. Schools had just reopened after the first lockdown and I had a bit more time to focus on training. It was time to take on Everest! One of my favourite running event companies Centurion were putting on a virtual challenge while events were still cancelled. Shifting the focus from distance to elevation, the challenge was to see how far you could climb in a week. Everest seemed like the perfect target. It leaned into my strengths and fitted my treadmill hiking experience perfectly. I always ran or hiked at an incline to lessen the impact on my body, using indoors sessions to push myself and outdoor runs to clear my head. By this stage, I hadn't raced for six months since the Country to Capital Ultra at the beginning of the year, and was desperate to sink my teeth into a new challenge.

The mental arithmetic was also appealing. Climbing 8848m on a treadmill while almost five months pregnant came with an array of logistical hurdles. I couldn't push my body to the limit, but I could find a way to adapt my target. Meticulous planning was required to meet my enhanced fuelling and hydration needs, and I needed to reconfigure my pacing strategy and posture to accommodate my bump. It was time to create a spreadsheet. Hiking on a cushioned treadmill seemed like the safest option for my problematic pelvis. I had a specialist machine that ramped all the way up to 40 per cent incline, much higher than gym treadmills that normally stop at 15 per cent. I knew when to suck up the pain of aching quads and when stabbing pains elsewhere meant I needed to rest. Like competing in an ultramarathon, I had to listen to my body carefully. I had to adapt. What my body could tolerate closely correlated to the treadmill incline setting. While I could raise it to 40 per cent incline my displaced centre of gravity meant this was not a wise – or safe – idea. I also wanted to keep my heart rate at around 140 beats per minute – elevated but not too high. My inner accountant was thrilled at the opportunity to crunch some numbers. I conducted an experiment to judge what incline I could tolerate on tired legs. The optimum climbing per heart rate beat was 20 per cent incline at 4.8km/h – the Goldilocks of hiking while pregnant.

Breaking it down into eight sessions over three days enabled me to balance work and kids with conquering the highest mountain in the world. There were a couple of work calls I had to make from the treadmill, and one of my last sessions was a family hike up local hills – the kids doing the equivalent elevation of Kinder Scout for their own Centurion medals. Combining a day out with the kids while ticking off some elevation was an ideal way to maximise my time. When it came to work, my colleagues understood that I was slightly bonkers and gracefully ignored my sweaty face breathing heavily down a video call, on occasions misting up the screen.

With a challenge like this I knew I needed to fuel correctly. I estimated eating 3500 to 4000 calories per day and got started on a food plan. This was going to be fun! Peering into the kitchen cupboards I reached back for the hidden stash of sour and fizzy Haribos – these would keep me smiling when climbing. The meal planner was filled with sweet treats from chocolate protein porridge, chocolate biscuits and my dad's homemade ice cream. My protein and carb fixes came from chicken and avocado sand-wiches, protein shakes, yoghurt, noodle stir fries and lasagne. And to replace my excessively salty sweat – which had contributed to my coma in Cambodia – I loaded up on salt and vinegar crisps and added the right amount of electrolyte tabs to my water.

I loved a puzzle and managing my posture was another prob-lem to solve. An eye-opening session with movement coach Shane Benzie the previous year had identified my imbalances. He quickly spotted which hip I carried the kids on, which caused me to slouch with my right hip outwards, reducing my elasticity. During this pregnancy I had suffered with some back ache, and I didn't want this to be exacerbated by climbing for nine hours. I stuck a note on the treadmill reminding me to stand tall – imagining a helium balloon was tied to my head pulling me skyward.

With the spreadsheet completed, the cupboards filled and Post-it notes strategically placed around the gym, I was ready to climb. Day one began as soon as I dropped the kids at school and nursery. Mounting the treadmill I was filled with excite-ment. Everest here I come! Within 10 minutes I was bored. The steady, monotonous pace didn't deliver the same mental stimulation as a varied interval session, and I wondered how on earth I was going to do it. Until now the tablet on the treadmill had been a superfluous accessory, but – Netflix to the rescue! – it finally proved its worth. Ninety minutes later I had climbed 1384m and learned about the crazy Italian game of calcio storico, a brutal mix of rugby and bare-knuckle boxing. Who knew climbing Everest could be so informative? Netflix episodes flew by thick and fast over the next three days as I soaked up every distraction possible.

My treadmill sessions varied from a swift 40 minutes to a mammoth 141, with gradients swinging between 16 and 20 per cent, depending on how tired my legs felt. During one evening session, John hopped on his bike alongside me, but quickly became absorbed in a Zwift competition that was beyond my comprehension. Life occasionally intervened – one hike was abruptly halted when an engineer turned up to fix our internet. Determined not to waste a training moment, I chatted to him while stretching my calves, casually hanging off the bottom step of the stairs. Sniffing the finish line, I took advantage of John doing school drop-off on the final morning, and set my sights on reaching the summit. Two hours and 21 minutes later I was done. I'd climbed Everest in less than 50 hours. I was relieved. I was proud. And a tiny part of me was sad it was over. But most of all I was delighted with how strong my body and mind were – just what I needed to take on labour and postpartum recovery.

On the back of this high I kept training consistently, even during a family break to the Brecon Beacons. One of the joys of trail running is being able to explore new locations and I had a new adventure before breakfast each day. While my back was sore (I may have extended a few drives with detours to get the relief from my heated car seat) I loved hiking with the family. Cormac even climbed Pen y Fan at two years and three months old, fuelled by Haribo. I was rising to the first crest of the rollercoaster again. It was not long before I came hurtling down.

I was pain free, 27 weeks pregnant and my boxing class was going brilliantly. I was wearing my beloved 16oz pink leather gloves which had thicker cushioning to reduce the impact from punches. Sliding on the musty cracked gloves was like being reunited with an old friend. I hadn't worn this heavier pair since my Muay Thai days in Thailand a decade ago, but right now they were just what I needed. Switching to floor work I moved into a series of weighted lunges, squats and a clean and press (lifting a weight from the floor to the shoulders then pushing it overhead). Failing to find a heavy enough weight on the rack I decided to add a twist to the bottom of the clean and press movement. Big mistake. I twisted to pick the dumbbell up at the start of the minute-long set and exploded upwards too quickly. Crunch, crunch, crunch. The top of my right hamstring pinged and I immediately knew something was wrong. The individual muscles of my hamstring felt oddly tangled up. Hoping it was just a small strain, I had a yummy protein shake at the gym to cheer myself up. Back at home while baking brownies I booked myself a physio appointment with Brett Davidson. I told myself it would be fine, but I just needed to double-check.

It was far from fine. I had probably torn my proximal hamstring, and Brett was worried the muscle might have ripped away from the bone. I had an uncomfortable pain in my butt and needed to see a sports consultant for my insurance to approve a scan. Things turned downhill from here. The specialist couldn't have been more dismissive of my injury. Since I was 28 weeks pregnant, he just didn't see why I needed to get back to training. Since I couldn't lie on my front or supposedly have an MRI (actually I could, since I was no longer in my first trimester), the tests he could do were limited, he said. At least he clarified the muscle had not come away from the bone. As far as this consultant was concerned, I should be sat on the sofa eating cake, allowing the injury to heal on its own. I tried to ask what I could do to aid recovery, but he was already standing up and ushering me out of the door. I felt invisible to him. I was not an athlete. I was just a baby carrier. I waddled back home trying not to cry.

With running out of the question – for a few weeks at least – I turned my attention to strengthening my arms and back, vital for carrying my newborn in a few months' time. Once more my training plans had changed, but I'd not given up on running. In fact, the run-in with the consultant made me even more determined to return. Brett luckily knew him, read him the riot act on how to treat female athletes and he finally authorised an MRI, which located the tear nowhere near his diagnosis. A bout of shockwave therapy and dry needling later, and the tensed-up muscles around my hamstring had loosened. At 31 weeks pregnant, I was given the go-ahead to start running again with a bit of tape to support my adductor. I dashed out into the pouring rain to try a gentle run-walk around a rugby pitch. I could still feel the tear, but was ecstatic to be able to move again. And besides, the soreness in my leg was nothing compared to the stitch created by the baby lying horizontally across my protruding belly. I tried to nudge her back into a more upright position, but she was having none of it. Never mind. It was time to enjoy my run in the rain.

As I entered my third trimester, I was insanely tired. The boys spent more time watching back-to-back cartoons, and at times I felt I was barely functioning. Often I found myself walking around in a daze brought on by sleep-disrupting stomach pains. I spent many moonlit nights doing laps of the bedroom and bathroom to try to ease the tension in my expanding belly. Compounding this was my inability to poo. I was backed up. Bouncing up and down running 20 miles a week had helped things along, so being injured had stopped more than one move-ment. Tiredness meant I wasn't always motivated to train and it felt like everything was grinding to a halt. The lows and highs of pregnancy continued as the weeks raced by, but as my due date approached, my mood lifted once more, and I started to feel primed for baby number three.

With just six weeks to go I was out running eight miles at a time, despite carrying an additional 9kg. My pelvic floor was under control and those shame-inducing second trimes-ter memories seemed a lifetime ago. Rest days at the weekends involved long hikes with the boys, who were now aged two and five, and I was riding the high of my newfound energy. I asked photographer Phil to capture this with a running pregnancy shoot at the top of my favourite hill, St Martha's on the North Downs Way. Unfortunately, it was short lived. Before long I was back to feeling every little stress and strain as my bump continued to expand. Each afternoon I would feel a hot poker sensation in the ribs. I spent hours walking around the house with a hot, microwaveable penguin tied to my back with a makeshift strap made from heart rate monitors. More missed training sessions. I needed another goal.

Less than two weeks before giving birth to Saoirse I embarked on a virtual half Ironman triathlon. ReRun, a charity ensuring running kit didn't go to landfill, had created an amusing challenge to keep endurance athletes occupied while races were cancelled. They received thousands of discarded race t-shirts every year and picked out 100 different races. You donated £10, then on a livestream a t-shirt would be picked for you at random, and you had to do the race on the t-shirt (however you interpreted it). I'm not sure what I was hoping for. I knew I wanted more than a 10k, but I was also aware I couldn't take on a 100-miler, even over a week. When my t-shirt was selected, a half Ironman seemed perfect.

I was aware that being this active while full-term pregnant was highly unusual. During my first pregnancy I could barely walk at this point as my son descended early, causing me to waddle around with the sensation of a head between my legs. Third time round and I was listening to specialist advice, training (mostly) well and seemed to be doused in a huge heap of my husband's Irish luck. The Everest attempt earlier in the year had taught me how to break down a task, so I took the same approach. Swimming pools were shut so the closest thing I could get to a water sport was our indoor rowing machine. The course was planned over five days and replicated the half Ironman distance. I was to row 1.9km, bike 90km and run a half marathon. Ever the mathematician I divided up my efforts:

days one and two centred on the row and cycle, day three was running part one, day four was pelvic floor recovery and day five finished off the 21.1km run.

The first dilemma was working out how to row with a small human growing inside me. My stomach was the size of a large beach ball and was getting in the way. Rather ungraciously, I had to spread my legs at the top of each pull to make way for my bump. It was a world away from my days on the Oxford college team merrily rowing the serene River Cherwell, chasing dates with fit young men. Here I was, a huge lump of a woman, locked indoors, pursuing a somewhat arbitrary goal in order to secure a chunk of metal on a ribbon. Chugging along at a bump-restricted speed limit, I completed the distance in a not too shabby 10 minutes. This was the easy part. Next, I had to work out how to get on to the bike.

Heaving myself into place I set off at a hard pace. Even this late in my pregnancy my competitive nature kicked in. Realising I might be overdoing it as my heart rate rose to 145 beats per minute, I eased off during the second hour. Powered by sweets I finished the 54km leg in two hours. I had to keep reminding myself that this was not a race, I had loads of time and I was about to give birth. After a self-inflicted pep talk, I eased off the next day. I tootled along on the bike keeping my heart rate at 125 beats per minute. Only now I couldn't get comfy. John's racing saddle was like sitting on a sharpened piece of wood, with my extra bump weight pressing me on to its hardened edges. I was also bored, bored, bored. Pedalling away at one speed for 36km without the variation of intervals was mind numbing. I was relieved when it was over, and so was my tender undercarriage.

Running at this point was putting additional strain on my pelvic floor and I knew I had to be sensible; I had to think about the long-term impact rather than the short-term goal. My idea of sensible was attempting 10.5km at a time with a rest day between. My idea of sensible was using a treadmill to lessen the impact and mixing up jogging and hiking. I really was listening to my body and making a conscious effort to keep my heart rate to 135 beats per minute. When the numbers on my monitor started to rise, I dialled back the speed. It was a constant recalibration based on the numbers.

Day four was a rest day. I needed to treat my pelvic floor with respect. So far it had been largely tolerating me, but it was time to give it a break. I didn't want to make it angry. Like any other muscle it got tired when overworked. Back-to-back days of running were not an option this late in my pregnancy, but that didn't mean I couldn't move. While the boys were at school, John and I went for a fast 10k hike, marching up the local hills. My sense of proportion was a little deluded, and viewing it as just a walk I forgot to take snacks. On the way home I started to feel dizzy. An afternoon on the couch protectively hugging the biscuit tin was the perfect recovery.

One day and six miles to go. I finished my half Ironman in style with a brilliant treadmill run. I alternated 10 minutes jogging at a 4 per cent incline and a speed of 9.2km/h with two minutes hiking at an 11 per cent angle and 5.6km/h pace. I was feeling strong again. I almost had to pinch myself. I was over 36 weeks pregnant.

Two weeks later and the clock was about to strike midnight. After hours of trying to get comfortable, contorting myself into different shapes around my pregnancy pillow, I had finally fallen asleep. Suddenly I woke up. The sheets were sodden and I was lying in a pool of faint pink liquid. What was going on? The baby wasn't due for more than a week and I'd convinced myself she was going to be late. It took me a moment to orientate myself. My waters had broken. Instinctively I grabbed my phone from the bedside cabinet and immediately called my parents, telling them to get in the car. Fortunately, they lived just 20 minutes away and were on standby to look after the boys.

John – where was John? Realising he was still downstairs watching a movie I shouted down to him, jolting him into action. Within 30 minutes we were at the maternity hospital. While the midwives checked me over in the sweltering ward,

John sat freezing in the car, Covid rules preventing him from coming in. Since I wasn't very dilated, I sent John to grab some sleep while I sat on the ward tapping on my TENS machine. The electrical pulses distracted me enough to manage the contraction pains, but within an hour the midwives told me to go home. I wasn't ready yet. With John not allowed in, I didn't feel safe and my body put labour on pause. Time to crack on with some work.

That same morning, I had a Women in Sport board strategy session. I was a trustee of the charity which campaigns for equal opportunities in British sport. Hiding my relatively mild contractions I joined at 9 a.m., failing to mention that I was in labour. By 10.30 a.m. I was talking less and less as the waves of contractions became stronger, cramping in my lower back and stomach. They were now around two minutes apart, but doggedly I carried on, determined to ensure I was contributing. When one contraction hit mid-speech, my Zoom gallery suddenly became a sea of concerned faces bearing down on me. I conceded it was time to go.

Calling ahead to the midwives, the birthing pool was full by the time we arrived. I was whisked straight into the delivery room and with every painful contraction started maxing out on the TENS machine. I sang out loud. Very loudly. Songs that would be on every 'motivational running' playlist. 'Bulletproof'. 'Stronger'. The same songs I carried in little plastic bags for the 246km of Spartathlon. The pain was intense, but unlike an ultra-marathon I knew it wouldn't last long. John was by my side giving me electrolytes, offering words of support. The perfect crew member. I entered the soothing water and grasped the gas and air. That stuff was brilliant. It was time to push. She was coming. As births go, it was a relatively smooth one, and fortunately Saoirse's head was smaller than those of her brothers. No need for stitches this time. Everything was going to plan. John captured a beautiful shot of the pair of us snuggling together, relaxed. It must have been quite the shock when the Women in Sport board, still wrapping up the strategy session, received the joyful photo of me and Saoirse. Proof that my abrupt departure had been entirely justified.

Coda: Be flexible

Through my pregnancy journey, I learnt the importance of flexibility. Initially confident about my exercise routine, reality soon challenged me. Experiencing unexpected setbacks like pelvic pain, bladder control issues and a severe hamstring tear taught me that rigid plans don't always align with the body's changing demands. Instead, adapting my training became essential. Embracing modifications, listening to professional guidance and responding to my body's signals allowed me to maintain fitness without compromising safety. When injuries halted running, I shifted focus to strength training; when outdoor activities felt uncomfortable, I relied on treadmill hikes. Accepting and adjusting to physical limitations during pregnancy not only kept me active, but strengthened my mindset, preparing me for labour and postpartum recovery. Ultimately, by learning to embrace the highs and lows and adapt accordingly, I experienced a happier, healthier and stronger pregnancy.

9
HAVE HOPE

From prolapse to the London Marathon

Emma's face was a mixture of shock and delight as I raised a 20-hour-old Saoirse to the webcam. She had been eight days early, and instead of a pre-labour pelvic health call we had skipped straight to the postpartum catch-up. Emma advised me to sleep as much as possible and 'awaken the area down there' – this was not the time to slack on my pelvic floor exercises. Food was her next concern. Was I eating enough? I recalled my post-labour nutrition with a wry smile: chocolate brownies, chocolate on toast, chocolate muffins. Calories were king. Healthy nutrition would have to wait.

Capturing the intimate conversation were Phil and Jon the videographers, camped out in my house just hours after I had given birth. Despite the intrusion I was keen to share my postpartum journey to show the reality – and possibility – of returning to running. Knowing I was keen to exercise as soon as humanly possible – without causing any long-term damage – Emma advised gentle treadmill walking within the first two weeks. But first I needed to pick up Donnacha from school. I had promised my six-year-old that I would collect him with his baby sister. He was keen to show her off to his friends, which meant I needed to hike the hill to school. A day after giving birth, with a swollen vagina, I was tackling that bloody hill again. I was pretty chuffed that walking didn't seem to be a problem despite soreness below.

And it was all worth it to see the look on Donnacha's face as his friends crowded around the buggy, cooing at his tiny new sister.

Hiking became part of my daily routine during Saoirse's first week. I walked for two hours at a time while she snuggled against me in the soft Caboo sling. Her delicate breath warmed my chest in the crisp winter air, and I felt grateful that I could move through the treasured landscape with her. But my emotions were torn. A week ago, I had been running powerfully on the tread-mill, and now my body was repatching itself following a massive trauma. My fitness had gone backwards. And I was starving all the time. Saoirse was a feeder, sucking liquid calories out of my body, cracking my nipples and destroying my energy. It felt like an immense step backwards.

John was the first to act. After a rough few days of endless feed-ing, he dragged me into the home gym. He could see I was never going to prioritise myself, the mum guilt weighing too heavily on my shattered mind, despite all I knew about the benefits. The moment I pressed start on the treadmill, I realised just how much I'd been missing that rush of endorphins. A jumbo smile spread across my face, and I ramped up the incline to 20 per cent. I was busting 170 beats per minute and breathing heavily. That first session was 6.4km of hiking at a pace of 6km/h. I stomped up 1000m of elevation and loved every second of it. I felt bloody brilliant. Yes, I would get a telling off from my coach for pushing too soon (and I did), but for those 60-odd minutes it was worth it. The foggy cloud lifted from my head and I had hope again.

Zombie status ruled for the next few weeks, as Saoirse refused to sleep for more than an hour at a time. Enforced rest became my norm – there simply wasn't a single moment to squeeze in a workout. I spent several evenings crumbled on the couch crying into Saoirse's muslins. While John was on the exercise bike upstairs, I was stuck on the sofa, Saoirse napping on me between feeds. I didn't want to watch TV. All I could think about was tidying the messy house and doing some stress-relieving stretches. I wanted to grab a glass of wine from the fridge instead of having a baby gnaw at my breast. I wanted to get my laptop and catch up with work.

I wanted to be anything other than a feeding machine. But I had been here before. Twice. And I knew it would pass. This was the low point and things would get better. I just had to give it time.

The game-changing moment came when I started pumping breast milk so John could do the 3 a.m. feed. Getting just a few hours of unbroken sleep helped me to survive the week and gave me the confidence – and time – to get back on the bike. At first, I was terrified of sitting on the tortuously hard seat, afraid it would be unbearable for my patchwork of healing skin, but as I tentatively lowered myself on to the bike, I was pleasantly surprised. No pain, just a slight numbness. It was time to see what I could do. Setting the bike to my pre-pregnancy power threshold I managed to hang on for the session, but my legs were absolutely dying. The freedom to go absolutely crazy with my heart rate was so liberating, but also very dangerous. I completely buried myself, feeding off the drug of endorphins, going all out. My body would never let me get to this intensity during pregnancy, always telling me, 'This is enough,' but now I had no self-limiter. Mentally I felt amazing, but my hamstring was not so forgiving. It was tight and unhappy. Now I had the dual battle of recovering from birth – and from injury. Deciding I needed to get my endorphin rush under control and take a more moderate approach, I opted to stick to treadmill hiking for the time being. Three hikes per week was winning. I didn't need to sweat my guts out on the bike.

Speaking to Eddie about my need to balance the desire for an exercise hit with a controlled recovery, she planned the sessions based on heart rate. They were just high enough to give me that amazing feeling at the end without busting myself in the process. Four weeks postpartum and I was having a follow-up call with Emma to determine next steps. I'd got back to exercise in the form of hiking, pelvic floor exercises and gentle stretching, but I wanted to gain strength. Emma gave me a list. Low-level core abdominal work was encouraged but I certainly wasn't ready for sit-ups or lifting weights above the head. The abdomen had to be protected at all costs, but I could use bodyweight, light weights and resistance bands for deadlifts, squats and hamstring curls.

Knowing my sleep-deprived brain would forget what to do, I stuck instructions on the gym wall. I was raring to go, but struggling to find time. If I missed Saoirse's reliable morning nap slot, I was too tired the rest of day to hit the gym. There was also the barrier of climbing two flights of stairs to the gym. I needed a different approach. I worked out what I could do in the kitchen while Saoirse played on her mat, and what I could manage when she was in the carrier. I did bits and pieces every day, often walking around the kitchen in funny poses, much to the amusement of two-year-old Cormac. My limbs grew stronger, but my pelvic floor was a different matter – I was still leaking when I stomped down the hill with the buggy. Cormac could now run faster than my powerwalk, and didn't understand why Mummy could no longer run with him. It was frustrating for Mummy too.

With so little time to train I began to slip back into the habit of chasing endorphins from cardio. I was rushing through my weight sessions, not taking the time to breathe properly and engage my pelvic floor. Instead, I was addicted to the heart rate increase, wanting every workout to feel hard. It was time to call Eddie, the voice of reason, again. During an emotional call Eddie told me I needed to focus on strength, but she was also acutely aware of my plummeting mental health and drive for the next endorphin hit. We discussed my running ambitions, and I described escaping to the fells and seeing the sun rise over the mountains having run through the night. That's what I was dreaming of.

We planned a local 50km ultra for six weeks' time (three months postpartum) as a training race before the Lakeland 100 miles. Saoirse would be seven months old by the time Lakeland 100 came round, and this seemed far more realistic than attempting UTMB three months after Cormac was born. I had already completed ten treadmill sessions, three bike workouts, lots of outdoor hiking and at least four strength sessions in the first six weeks of Saoirse's life. It felt like I was doing nothing, but I had to accept it was a gradual process. I couldn't run just yet. My body was stuck in limbo. I was no longer pregnant, but neither was I back to full strength. Far from it. Seeing my giggling boys race down the hill as we headed out the front door was becoming increasingly bittersweet. I desperately wanted to chase after them, but had to reach the next milestone first: my six-week check.

There was a lot riding on my face-to-face appointment with Emma. It was a mummy MOT to measure the effects of pregnancy and labour, and I was banking on it being the green light to start running again. As I entered Emma's examination room I was feeling upbeat. This time felt different. I had no pain in my pelvis and although I had been leaking in the first few weeks this had eased off considerably. With a mask covering most of her face Emma asked me to hop up on to the doctor's couch. She began by prodding my tummy – apologising for her cold fingers – to see what kind of gap I had in my abdomen. This is normal after pregnancy and every woman's gap is a different size. Mine was not too bad, but there was still a lot to do. So far, so OK.

The next stage was a series of strength movements to gauge how much internal pressure was being placed on my stomach muscles. I successfully performed a press-up and plank on the inclined couch before squatting, bending and twisting. My upper back was stiff from hunching over while breastfeeding, and Emma, never one to mince her words, announced that I had 'general global weakness'. This was not going so well. I really needed to strengthen my glutes and pelvis to start running decent distances again.

We then moved on to pelvic floor tests, where I hopped and jumped about in the small examination room, trying to avoid the furniture. At six weeks postpartum Emma was not surprised to find my bladder was still leaking. This was all normal and she expected to see a lot of improvement in the coming weeks. This gave me hope.

But things took a hard left turn after my internal examination. Placing a surgical glove over her hand, Emma inserted her finger inside me to feel my pelvic floor muscles. There was good news. My pelvic floor was working and all my squeezes while boiling the kettle were paying off. Asking me to stand up, Emma checked again. This time the news was not so good. I couldn't fully engage the muscles at the back, and nothing was happening at the front. Shocked, I gasped audibly when Emma told me I had a prolapse.

The front wall of my uterus had slipped down from its normal position into the vagina. It was classed on a scale of one to four with four being the most severe. Mine was a two, with the back wall a one. I was not expecting this. I had no symptoms – other than a weak pelvic floor, which I'd had before. I thought prolapse happened to post-menopausal women, not to fit, strong women in their late thirties. Emma had a different viewpoint. Having had three babies and done an inordinate amount of running, it was more surprising that I hadn't had a prolapse until now. More than half of women with two or more children have one, except most just don't know. I realised it was incredibly common, but no-one talked about it. Women don't necessarily recognise the symptoms or get them checked out. We just carry on. Once more, I felt women's health was being ignored.

Emma gave me a firm warning. If I wanted to be running in 10 years' time, I had to hold off right now. Running now could cause irreversible damage further down the line. I needed to re-evaluate my goals. I would not be running 50km in five weeks' time. I didn't know when I'd be running again. Would I ever run again? This wasn't supposed to happen. I'd done everything right. Listened to every expert I could. This wasn't what I wanted. It wasn't what I expected, but I was going to play the cards I'd been handed as well as I could. I couldn't control what had happened, but I could control how I reacted to it.

The consultation with Emma was just the wake up call I needed. It was time to forget about heart rate and rewire my brain. I needed to focus on slow, purposeful strength workouts, breathing correctly to squeeze my pelvic floor. The session took an hour – a huge chunk out of my already stretched day – but it was better to do half the session correctly than rush through the whole thing. If I got this right, I would be able to run again. It was back to lunges across the kitchen floor as I emptied the dishwasher, singing 'The Wheels on the Bus' to Saoirse as she lay on her play mat.

I was lucky enough to be able to afford Emma's support and knew she was working for my best interests. Disappointingly, I couldn't say the same about my local GP. Yet again I was viewed as a vessel for a baby rather than a person in my own right. At my eight-week GP check, I answered her closed questions honestly and in full. I raised concerns about my mental health and how the lack of structured training was impacting me. I said it more than once, but she didn't really hear me. She glanced up briefly, told me to 'do my exercises' and handed me a generic leaflet. That was it. No questions about how I was coping. No discussion of what support I might need. No recognition of how hard it is to go from feeling strong and active to suddenly being stuck, and the impact it might have on my ability to be the best mother I could. Just a quick box-tick about contraception – as if that was the most pressing thing in my world. Apparently, the fact that I was going to the toilet and was able to walk meant I was 'fine'. Saoirse was healthy, so there was nothing else to discuss. I felt dejected and invisible. Once again, I cried on the way home.

Salvation came a few weeks later in a most unexpected form – a block of silicone. This was the pivotal moment, the last piece of the puzzle on the road to recovery. A pessary. I was accustomed to wearing a knee support, having injured it in the past, and now I needed a support for my undercarriage. I was in rehab after all. On Emma's recommendation I visited former Great Britain rower Tracey Matthews for an assessment. Tracey worked as a pelvic health pessary specialist and her elite sport background meant she really understood my needs. This wasn't just about getting back to everyday life pain- and leak-free, it was about being able to run high-impact ultramarathons. Upon arrival Tracey opened a box of rubber items. The pessaries came in a range of shapes and sizes – some rings, others more cube-like. It was a whole new world. I had no idea these things existed. She had a feel of my prolapse, then pulled out a silicon cube and handed it to me to insert. I slid behind the curtain and slotted it inside. It felt surprisingly comfortable – like a tampon with suckers made of medical grade silicon.

Tracey asked me to jump up and down before sending me out to run the streets. She wanted to test the device in my natural environment, to measure the stress my body would face.

It was the first time I'd run since giving birth and I was ecstatic. Finally, I was allowed to run! As I headed down White Hart Lane, I pulled into a faster stride, lifting my feet over potholes and cracked paving. Climbing over the railway bridge stairs and back down the other side I felt incredible. Suddenly I didn't have to worry about leaking. The little cube of plastic – which looked alarmingly like a baby teething toy – was absolute genius. I just had to make sure it didn't get mixed up with Saoirse's ones.

I reached home elated. My prolapse was not fixed, but my symptoms were considerably improved. Hope was on the horizon and I could visualise myself running towards it. Aware that I had to keep myself under control, I made a promise to wear the pessary for long hikes only and not to run before the sign-off from Emma. After the shock of discovering the prolapse I now felt armed with knowledge, a strength plan and my new best friend – Poppy the pessary.

Poppy went everywhere with me. She was the best secret accessory in the world. At two months postpartum I was finally given the go-ahead to slowly return to running – with Poppy by my (in)side. Beginning with 20-second steep hill reps on the soft trail, the following day I was able to run at a slow pace on soft ground for seven minutes. I built up my time and distance over the next four weeks, managing a one-hour soft trail run at three months postpartum. While heavily pregnant with Saoirse I had been doing hour-long runs quite happily, and now it had taken me three months to return to that point. Three years ago, I had been competing at UTMB just three months after giving birth to Cormac, but this recovery had been completely different. I was nowhere near that level of fitness or healing. It had never dawned on me that my recovery would take so long. My plans – documented by our film – to run 50k at three months postpartum had gone completely out of the window.

My perspective on running had to shift. I needed to learn how to become a social runner, so I started running with friends, using it as time to enjoy myself rather than training to race. Through my social runs, I gradually built up my ability to withstand uphill and flat trails, concrete and – hardest of all – running downhill leak-free. What shocked me most wasn't the immediate effect that Poppy had, but the lack of knowledge amongst other mothers. As I shared my story with my running mums, on my blog and on my Instagram feed, people reached out, telling me they never knew pessaries were a solution for prolapse. It was not covered in prenatal training. It was not part of postpartum support. Other mums were not talking about it. Once more, women's needs were being underserved and our goals ignored. A tiny piece of silicon changed everything for me. After childbirth, I felt lost in my own body – leaking, weak, ashamed – and no one was talking about it. A pessary gave me back the confidence to run, to feel strong again. It was shocking how something so small could make such a big impact, yet there was no investment to educate or support women to find these solutions after doing the most powerful thing in the world: bringing life into it.

With my 50k race off the cards – and the film ending with me running with my local mum friends instead – I turned my attention to another virtual race. I had enjoyed the half Ironman in lockdown, and the ability to interpret a challenge any way you liked. I loved having a goal to focus on, but didn't want to be pushing hard in a race. This time the random selection pulled out the Humber Half Marathon. This was 13.1 miles across 13 bridges in the northeast of England. Down south in Surrey I replicated this by running under or over 13 bridges, many of them along the River Wey. I finished in 2:10, my first two-hour run since having Saoirse. I was still a long way off my 43-hour UTMB run three months postpartum with Cormac, but I was making progress.

On 1 May, five months postpartum, I ran a 50km ultra. It might sound impressive, but the real feat wasn't the running, it was the logistics of fitting it into family life. The race was close to home and took me just under five and a half hours. That extra half hour? Breastfeeding. I'd pumped before heading out in the morning, but halfway through the race I had to feed Saoirse. To make it work, John had to get both boys to their multisport club and bring Saoirse to meet me at an exact spot, within a tight 15-minute window. I had to pace the first half perfectly so we could rendezvous in the car park, latch her on, and leave enough time for John to swing back to collect Cormac. It was like coordinating a military operation. Looking back, it was mad. At the time I remember thinking, what on earth are we doing? But John made it back in time to pick up Donnacha from the longer multisport session and even get to the finish line, so the boys could run in with me. It was chaotic, precise, hilarious – and completely normal for our version of family life.

Next up was the Lakeland 100. This was far more than just a race for me. It was personal. My late grandmother had lived in the Lake District, and the region held so many childhood memories – our family holidays were spent scrambling over rocks, wading through icy rivers and getting soaked by surprise downpours. It was my grandmother who gave me that adventurous spark, as well as a drive to help others. In her eighties she was still volunteering, serving tea with the Red Cross, and had an energy that never seemed to run out. As a child I utterly adored her, and in adulthood I realised how much of her feisty spirit lived on in me, as it does now in Saoirse. She revelled in telling stories of her past, planting the seeds of independence and adventure that would shape my life. It wasn't until years later that I found out she'd also been a brilliant cross-country runner. Somehow, it made sense. And it made me want to honour her with this race; to run not just for me, but for her too.

Saoirse was now seven months old and I only had time for a quick adventure. I travelled up by train with Matt trying to pump breastmilk along the journey. We were barely off the train before Matt realised he couldn't find our tent poles and we'd have nowhere to sleep pre- or post-race. Cue panic. He was spiralling, imagining the race ruined before it had begun. I switched into calm mum mode. It was second nature now. When you're a mum, there's no time for flapping. Something worse is always round the corner. I asked the right questions, retraced our steps and began prepping a plan B to crash in the organiser's marquee. Within an hour, they were found. Crisis averted.

During the race briefing I stood in the crowd with two wireless breast pumps stuck inside my sports bra. I was determined to drain as much milk as possible before setting off, and new technology made that far easier than before. Once the race began, it was all about managing myself over the long haul and managing my milk supply. I had to carry a pump and stop at various points to express milk. There were no private spaces, no designated areas, just whatever patch of trail or checkpoint I could find. People stared. I felt uncomfortable and undignified. I also wasted a huge amount of time trying to trigger my let-down reflex in the cold, noisy checkpoints. I remember crouching in a tent, willing the milk to come, watching a video of Saoirse crying on my phone, trying to fool my body into thinking she was there. I needed the video to make the milk flow. That moment hit me hard. I realised how little provision there was for mums like me at races. The logistics of expressing on the move had never been thought through – because no one had ever expected a breastfeeding mother to be doing this.

And then, in the middle of the night, something else shook me. I was running alone in the dark when I noticed a man slot in on the narrow path right behind me. He didn't pass. He didn't speak. He just stayed there, uncomfortably close, striding step in step with me. I asked him several times if he wanted to go ahead – but he didn't respond. It was intimidating. I didn't feel in danger, exactly, but I felt trapped. I sped up just to get some distance. It was another moment that made me pause. Men don't often realise the positions women find themselves in during these races – isolated, exposed, watched. It's an additional level of mental strain men never have to carry.

However, despite the discomfort, the exhaustion, and the obstacles, I never once considered quitting. I couldn't. I didn't have time to come back and try again. This was my only shot. And the kids were waiting to see my medal, which luckily was big and sparkly. It was also proof that mum did what she said she would. I finished the 100 miles in 33 hours. Not the fastest, but solid. I could still hike well and that made all the difference in the latter stages. There was no grand celebration at the end – just a quick shuffle to the station and a train ride home – and I immediately slipped back into family life as if I hadn't just run through two days and nights across the fells. But it meant something. It meant I could still do hard things, still take on adventures. And in my own quiet way I'd honoured the woman who first showed me how. It had also taught me motherhood was not the finish line; it was just another checkpoint.

I'd always known that if I was ever going to draw a line under my postpartum recovery, it wouldn't be in a clinic or by being signed off with a medical form. It would be on tarmac. I decided to run the October 2021 London Marathon as the ultimate pelvic floor test. Nothing quite proved readiness like pounding 26.2 miles of unforgiving road. I'd avoided road marathons all my running life. They never appealed. I'd skipped building up distances and PBs, and jumped straight into the big guns of running ultras. When my running friends signed up for big city races, all they seemed to care about was beating their personal best (PB). I'd ask them what they saw along the route – the architecture, the culture, the feel of the place and they'd just shrug. 'Didn't notice,' they'd say, 'but I shaved 30 seconds off my PB.' That was never me. I wanted to feel the run. Experience the place. Share smiles with strangers on muddy climbs. Tarmac always felt too sterile, too artificial, but this time was different. I needed the road and a definitive test. I needed to know my body, after everything, could go the distance on hard, flat ground without pain or damage.

Even before the race began, I had a taste of what it meant to be a woman trying to return to sport. I wasn't allowed to take 10-month-old Saoirse with me to the race expo to collect my bib. No children were permitted in the vast exhibition hall. I had to scramble to sort childcare just to pick up a race number. That experience stayed with me. It was my first real experience of how the London Marathon – like so much of sport – still created barriers for women; barriers which sent the message, 'This space wasn't built with you in mind. You don't belong.'

It was a similar feeling the next day as I stood penned in my corral surrounded by a sea of carbon-plated men. Where were all the women? Despite the uneasiness of standing chest to back with a heap of male runners inside I felt calm. I wasn't chasing a time. I was chasing a feeling: control, strength, ownership. I wanted my body to be mine again, not something I feared or worked around. I wanted to run free.

The gun went off, the miles clicked by, and I was buoyed by the crowds along the route, and strangers who recognised me and shouted my name. Pace was irrelevant, I ran to feel. My pelvic floor held strong. My legs felt sure. My heart was full. Hope had pulled me through. I crossed the finish line in 3:23 and burst into tears. I was absolutely elated. I had done it. For the first time in nearly a year, I felt fully me. I had closed a chapter. I wasn't broken anymore. I wasn't recovering. I was back. And I'd proved it, mile by mile, on the one surface I used to avoid.

I didn't realise it at the time, but the London Marathon would become a major turning point for me – in more ways than one. While I had been privately battling to be race ready, I was fighting on another front with the race director. I hadn't been looking for a fight – it had simply landed in my DMs. In May 2021, as I was still struggling with my own return to running, a message landed in my Instagram inbox from a runner named Jess Welborn. She was in a difficult position – one I knew all too well – and I couldn't ignore it. Jess had worked incredibly hard to qualify for a Championship place in the 2021 London Marathon. It's a category that sits just below the elite field, reserved for top-tier amateur and club runners. She'd run a blistering 2:52 marathon in 2020, well under the 3:14 qualifying time, but she was now pregnant, due just eight weeks before race day. She asked London Marathon if she could defer. The answer was no.

This was a different scenario to my own situation with UTMB. At the time of my 2018 race no one was allowed a pregnancy deferral, but London Marathon was different. Those with a ballot place could defer (albeit only for a year – SheRACES guidance would ask for at least two years), but the faster runners in the Championship or Good for Age entry could not. London Marathon's policy was clear: no deferrals under any circumstances. Illness, injury, pregnancy, jury duty – it didn't matter. Their rigid qualification windows left no room for life events, even ones that disproportionately affected women. It made no sense. Their refusal was forcing women to either lose their hard-earned place or risk returning to running too soon postpartum – often before it was medically safe. Jess was told she could either run the marathon at eight weeks postpartum or she could qualify again by running a 1:28 half marathon before year's end at just four months postpartum. It wasn't just unfair – it was discriminatory.

I wrote to London Marathon, sharing Jess's story. I explained the risks of returning too early. I referenced studies showing that many women return stronger a year after birth if they're given the right time and support; returning too soon could lead to long-term damage. I argued that offering deferrals wasn't a concession, it was equality of opportunity. The reply from London Marathon was polite but firm: Championship places couldn't be deferred for any reason. They dug in, failing to see that the rules themselves were part of the problem. Their argument was that the longer the time that had passed since you'd had achieved the qualification time, the less likely you were to repeat it. Which made sense, unless you'd had a baby in the meantime and needed time to recover. Jess would have been far more likely to repeat her qualification performance at eight months postpartum than eight weeks (this was the post-Covid year of two London marathons being held in a year, which also made matters more complicated).

Their model treated men and women the same, but that wasn't equitable. Equal rules did not give men and women the same opportunities. Equality was not the same as equity. It was ignorance. Women weren't small men. And maternity wasn't a 'choice' that should cost someone their place on the start line. When logic and polite private correspondence didn't work, I had no option but to turn to visibility. I reached out to *The Telegraph* and *Women's Running*. Jess's story hit the headlines. The response was overwhelming. Women messaged me and Jess with their own experiences, thanking us for speaking up, and many more revealed they'd been quietly denied too. Some hadn't even bothered to ask for deferrals, having heard through clubs that it wasn't allowed. The issue wasn't just about Jess, it was about all women. Still, London Marathon wouldn't budge. I had a call with the senior leadership team, joined by Jess. We hoped they would come up with solutions. Instead, we were told only two women were affected, so this wasn't really an issue, but we knew from our correspondence alone that this figure was wrong. One of the London Marathon team even claimed he personally understood what it took to return to fitness after childbirth because he'd seen his wife do it twice. Jess and I were speechless. London Marathon then told *The Telegraph* that Jess was 'not really asking for deferral but rather that she should be allowed to qualify for a 2022 Championship place based on a performance achieved outside the designated qualification window.' Instead of the simple option of supporting mothers back to the start line, they seemed set on denying us.

But the tide was turning. Another runner, Kelly Stokes, had the idea (and contacts) to appeal to London Marathon's sponsor, Virgin Money, who quickly confirmed that of course deferrals should be allowed. That pressure worked. Quietly, London Marathon changed their stance. Pregnant and postpartum women would now be allowed to defer, but only to a general entry. No Championship or Good for Age. And they still had to pay again. London Marathon also refused to announce the change publicly. So I did. I shared it widely, using the platform my UTMB photograph had given me, and I made sure women knew they could ask.

Eventually, in July 2022, the deferral option was officially extended so Championship and Good for Age runners could race from the start lines they had earned. It was a step forward, but even now women must still pay again for another entry after having a baby – something I'm still fighting against. What looked like a victory quickly revealed itself as only scratching the surface, highlighting a systematic problem within the world of racing. Too often, progress is presented as equality when in reality it's closer to gender-washing. Organisations proudly sign declarations like Brighton plus Helsinki, committing to equity for women in all they do, and brands talk endlessly about inclusion – yet many still sponsor events that don't deliver it.

For the London Marathon, women can technically defer if they become pregnant, but they must pay again to run – and at other London Marathon events there's no deferral at all. On the surface it looks like progress, but dig into the detail and it falls far short of true equity.

Standing at the London Marathon expo, unable to bring my newborn inside to collect my race bib, I felt the weight of it all. The policy battles, the dismissals, the restrictions – they weren't just about pregnancy. They were part of a wider pattern. Sport, even something as seemingly inclusive as running, wasn't built with women in mind. I realised that the barriers weren't just about safety on the trails, breastfeeding spaces, t-shirt sizing or deferral policies, they were structural, cultural, baked into the way races were designed and delivered. And I couldn't unsee it. I knew something had to change. And I knew I couldn't wait for someone else to do it. It had to be me.

Coda: Have hope

After giving birth to Saoirse, I clung to hope, not just for my body to heal, but for change in the sport I loved. My recovery was anything but smooth: a prolapse diagnosis, endless pelvic floor exercises and months of doubt. But I kept going, determined to run again. At the same time, I was quietly battling the London Marathon. Through tears, pain and endless pelvic floor exercises, I kept going. And when I finally crossed the finish line of my first road marathon, I knew I was back. Hope carried me through injury, exhaustion and bureaucracy. I believed in my body and I believed in the power of change. I still do. Because women deserve better and sometimes the most powerful thing you can do is force the world to notice.

10

YOU BELONG

24 Hour Championships, Italy and Taiwan

The baby-shaped pause button had been lifted. For the first time in nearly a decade I wasn't trying to get pregnant, pregnant or recovering from pregnancy. There was no rush to fit in a race before the next baby arrived. Our family was complete. I'd always known Saoirse would be my last child. After Cormac, I would continue to coo at babies, but after child number three the gnawing maternal ache completely disappeared. Donnacha and Cormac were so different from each other, always bouncing between companionship and competition, but when Saoirse came along it was like she completed the triangle. It was the three of them, a little ecosystem that just made sense. The jostling for attention eased. The energy between them balanced. We were whole.

But with that wholeness came something unexpected: space. Mental space, emotional space and physical space too. I could start thinking beyond the next nap, feed or school run. After the London Marathon, I felt physically strong again. Not just holding-it-together strong. Managing my prolapse was no longer the daily battle it had been. I no longer constantly thought about leaking during my runs, and started not to need my pessary for shorter, softer trail runs, which felt like a massive step forward. For the first time in years I had the mental and physical capacity to really go after something big. But what should it be?

Everything came together at the Maverick South Downs 54km trail race in November 2021. I wasn't just ticking over anymore. I was in the top 12 per cent of all runners, coming second female in 5:31:25. A few years earlier I had only been around the top 25 per cent. I could immediately see a huge improvement and I wanted to capitalise on it. Speaking to my coach Eddie, we started a process of 'dating my goals'. It was important to select the right goal, and every goal was going to be a massive commitment. I started thinking about each goal in depth, one by one, and considering what it would mean. I called this dating because I felt like I was having chats with each goal and thinking about what a future would be like together. And it wasn't just about the race, it was about the life that came with training for it. How would it fit with family life? Would I enjoy the process or just grind through it for a finish line photo? What would it mean to me to achieve this goal? I needed to be excited about the journey, not just the result.

I broke up with some goals fairly quickly. A parkrun PB? I didn't care. A sub three-hour marathon? Too much volume, not enough trails. I'd be on roads all the time, away from the places that actually brought me joy. Also, I'd seen the stress that chasing marathon PBs had caused many of my friends. But I'd also already had my share of 'just finish' challenges. I'd done numerous multi-stage races in amazing locations around the world. I didn't want to tick another box just to say I'd done it. Mountain races like Tor des Géants weren't my strength either. Too much technical terrain, too slow and I couldn't be competitive. I wanted the race to be about my fitness rather than my technique. I was craving something long and hard, that played to my strengths. I wanted to get back to − or perhaps for the first time consider more seriously − performance.

That's when Spartathlon came back into focus. I'd done it before, but only just finished. I knew I could do better. It was a long, tough road race. No tree roots or rocks to trip on. The conditions were brutal, but it was consistent, steady. It was about pacing, management, strength over time. I visualised myself arriving at the statue of Leonidas in Spartathlon, my boys cycling beside me at the end alongside the locals. I wanted a second stab at it, to test myself and improve my result. To do myself justice. To finally go from pregnancy to performance. But first, I had to qualify.

From the start, I didn't just want to scrape into the ballot. I wanted certainty, to earn an automatic qualifying place by going beyond the minimum. The standards were brutal but clear: for women, running 170km in 24 hours got you into the ballot, but reaching 212.5km – at a pace of 6:47 minutes per kilometre – got you a golden ticket and automatic qualification into the British squad. It seemed possible. I didn't want to risk missing out. There were multiple ways to qualify, from running 12 hours up to 48 hours, on flat terrain or in the mountains. If you were 25 per cent better than the standard time (set for each distance) then you had an automatic qualification, whether that was over a 12-hour race or 24-hour race. I analysed the numbers and paces needed, and selected 24 hours as the optimal distance for being '25 per cent better' than the standard and gaining that auto qualifier. I needed to do it in the most straightforward way, so I opted for a 24-hour track race where I knew I could eliminate terrain and logistical variables and perform at my best. I picked Phoenix Track Wars in Walton-on-Thames. It was close to home, low key and logistically simple.

Training went smoothly – once I sorted my period out. It had still not returned 15 months after having Saoirse. I was still breastfeeding – as she had several food allergies I was painstakingly desensitising her to – so I was eating enough calories overall to keep up my milk supply, but my workouts were unknowingly under-fuelled. Research shows that eating erratically throughout the day affects women's performance more than it affects men's. The stress of juggling three kids, advocacy work, freelancing and board meetings meant I was often eating late at night, meaning I was literally running on empty during the day. I made a conscious effort to adjust my eating schedule, eating more calories at lunchtime and shifting dinner to a more civilised time. I stopped breastfeeding as Saoirse weaned further and John took over her early morning feed, so I could get more sleep and recover from training. The additional sleep and change in mealtimes helped my period to return. I have always judged the health of my body by the regularity of my cycle, so I was relieved when I started to menstruate again and had a monthly marker to tell me my body was in balance.

Unfortunately, I didn't take the same sensible approach to my race taper (cutting down miles and intensity in the lead up to a race to rest your body and mind) as the day of my attempt approached. With a drop in training hours, I thought it was a great opportunity to catch up on family admin. A mountain of dentist appointments, baby gear donations, kids' shoe shopping and haircuts filled my days leading up to the race. I arrived at the start line already tired from life – I was not mentally recovered from the tough training.

As I lined up on the familiar eight-lane red track at 9.a.m. the wind buffeted my curly locks. It was a motley crew of random runners, all with their own goals. Some were aiming to see how far they could walk in 24 hours while others were hoping to hit 100km – before calling it a day. The event was designed to be flexible with some chasing time goals and others seeking a specific distance. As a result, it was an even mix of women and men, no one feeling under pressure because there were no cut-offs to hit. You simply ran what you could.

I was aiming to run for 24 hours non-stop and had three goals in mind. The A goal was to automatically qualify for Spartathlon (by running 212.5km), the B goal was to run over 200km, and the C goal was to qualify for the Spartathlon ballot by running 170km.

John and I decided that he would crew for me during the race, as it would be good preparation for Spartathalon. He had no real clue what he was doing, but was enthusiastic, nonetheless, and knew better than anyone how to motivate me to keep going when things got tough, as they inevitably would. Luckily my friend Alison Walker was also running (she was attempting to set a Malaysian record) and her husband was a pro at crewing for her. I'd met Alison on a night ultra in 2019 and we had bonded over our shared love of running for a very long time. John tagged on to Alison's husband, learning the ropes, and immediately regretted not thinking about bringing a shelter to have a nap in, or at least a chair to sit on to watch the laps pass by.

I was also clueless. Perhaps it was the bounciness of track or the joy of knowing there was nothing to stumble over, but I set off too fast. I covered the first 16km at a five minute per kilometre pace – a classic rookie error.

Fuelling was also a fast learning curve. John stood by the side of the track waving to attract my attention before handing me food as I ran past. I was accustomed to eating on the move so continued to run as I took on fuel. John initially tried to stuff me full of 400 calories an hour, but we soon realised this was too much. Bars didn't go down well and Pringles were the only real food I could stomach. I tried to ignore John, refusing to catch his eye because I couldn't face anymore food. In hindsight, jam sandwiches would have been perfect – they became a staple in later races – but we hadn't discovered their magic yet. Switching to gels helped my stomach settle down and I eased into the race. Perhaps too much. I became so relaxed that I started chatting to other runners and slowing down to run alongside them. By this point there were still a few dozen runners, which gave me plenty of opportunity to natter on the 400m track. John – who was under strict instructions from Eddie to get bossy when he needed to – told me off for chatting. I needed to stick to my own pace. Time to knuckle down. Sticking in my earphones I put on a David Goggins audiobook, chuckling to myself while trying to stay focused. As I ran into the night I moved to music to help keep the rhythm of my pace: classic nineties cheesy pop – anything I knew the lyrics to that could keep my brain functioning.

The event also included three separate six-hour races, designed so people could technically run three separate marathons in a 24-hour period and increase their total in a bid to join the 100 Marathon Club (or just run a marathon after work or at midnight). This meant much faster runners joined every now and then, with others dropping out, which was slightly off-putting to start with, but at least changed the scenery of bodies. John took a quick nap before dawn, as I could fuel from the communal aid station for a while, and I needed him focused for the important last hours.

As the end of the race approached early on Saturday morning, I started to struggle. My pace was slipping and I kept getting stuck behind a trio in fancy dress walk-running three abreast, refusing to leave a small gap on the inside, as track etiquette would dictate. 'I'm not moving for her,' said one of the women, which surprised me as I've always found ultrarunning a supportive community. Every time I had to run the bend in lane four, I lost vital seconds. It was going to be tight. The line between making the auto-qualifier and just missing out was becoming thinner. A long toilet stop could derail me at any time.

Eventually I plucked up the courage to push my way past on the inside, trying my best not to let out my inner track-rage. I made it through to the finish with 1.1km to spare, running 213.6km. I wasn't really aware I was first overall. It hadn't registered because I was just aiming for a distance. I had my goal and wherever I came in the standings didn't matter. There was no trophy, but I felt justified in sneaking a few extra Freddos from the food table to take home to the kids.

I was desperate to sleep and recover, but first we had to deal with the children. We had made a major parenting error. John, like me, was shattered. He'd napped briefly in the car during the night, but was mostly running on fumes. We drove home in a fog, arriving back around 11 a.m. (we would always nap before driving now – sleep deprivation has a big impact on reaction times). My parents had been looking after the kids, but left as soon as we arrived, their promised duty complete. Donnacha was unimpressed that I had no trophy for coming first for his show-and-tell – and I shared his sentiment. But most of all I just wanted to sleep. Except we had three small children to entertain and we were both severely sleep deprived. The next eight hours were an utter mess as we tag-teamed naps and tried to stay upright, the house a chaos of overexcited children and exhausted adults. But it didn't matter. My dream had been realised. I was going to Sparta.

Just days after I finished my race, everything changed. I got a message from Robbie, my former coach who was part of the management for the Great Britain 24-hour team. While I'd been focused on automatically qualifying for Spartathlon I'd simultaneously – and unwittingly – hit the qualifying distance for Team GB. Robbie asked if I would like my name to be put forward for the European Championships in Verona. The caveat? It was in the same month as Spartathlon. I had been so desperate to kiss that statue again, but the thought of wearing a GB vest completely shifted my focus. This wasn't just about me, it was the story. The fairy-tale transformation from being second-last in the school mile to running for my country. I knew how powerful that could be, especially for women and girls like me – the ones who never saw themselves as athletes and who still shied away from taking part in sport, burdened by painful memories. There was something else too. I found I loved the camaraderie of racing for a team and running for others rather than myself. I'd run a club race for Guildford and Godalming in October 2021 and loved chasing points for something bigger than me. It was the first time I'd ever made an effort for a sprint finish. That's what Verona offered. A chance to be part of something and to show other women there's a different way to belong in sport. Spartathlon could wait.

The next five months were a whirlwind of training, racing and advocacy. Yet my imposter syndrome kept festering away. Intrusive thoughts – 'I'm not an elite athlete. I'm just a runner. I'm not a professional' – kept sneaking into my head like an unwelcome trespasser, attempting to steal nuggets of confidence. Fortunately, my life was so hectic I didn't have time to dwell on self-doubt.

A month after the track event, I was racing in a local 40-miler. I had completely forgotten about the Fox Ultra until the event details pinged into my inbox. Once more my racing strategy was dictated by family needs. I had a 15-minute window to reach the finish line and secure my lift home. It was the only window John had between kid pickups. If I missed that opportunity I would be walking an additional four miles. We were a one car household, and John needed the vehicle to collect the kids from clubs. I raced with purpose – getting a lift – and finished second female, but still no trophy. I made a mental note to only enter races that had them so Donnacha wouldn't complain again.

Spring and summer brought with them a slew of races as I trained hard ahead of Verona. Eddie continued to coach me, and helped me plan a summer of races which balanced fun with pushing myself. She knew that enjoying my running always led to the best outcomes. I took in the beauty of the Isle of Mull during the Impact Marathon, alongside planting trees and dancing ceilidhs after the race. I made it round the South Downs Way 100-miler in well under 20 hours, perfectly timed to tag John so he could leave for his cycling sportive the next day. On the roads I pushed the pace at the Big Half, a half-marathon around four London boroughs, running under 90 minutes after a big training week. Poppy the pessary came along for every long run, but I was finally strong enough to leave her behind on the shorter ones. And just as my running confidence was gaining strength, so was my voice.

Since leaving my job in 2019, alongside new work projects I had dedicated much of my time to equality in sport. I sat on the board of Women in Sport, was an ambassador for the Active Pregnancy Foundation, and was working behind the scenes with races around the world to level up their policies. The photograph at UTMB had been the catalyst for all manner of change in my life. Coming at just the right time, as we were planning to move out of London, it had flipped my career from making profits for shareholders to advocating for women in sport.

In April 2022 I found myself walking through the Saatchi Gallery, slightly dazed and utterly humbled. My UTMB breast-feeding photo was featured in the *In-Focus: Women's Sport through the Lens* exhibition. It was surreal. This wasn't just a collection of race snaps or medals on walls. It was a celebration of the most powerful moments in women's sport from the last 50 years; images that had sparked global conversation, broken the inter-net and shifted perspectives. My photo sat between two legends: Jamaican Shelly-Ann Fraser-Pryce, one of the greatest sprinters of all time, and Dame Sarah Storey, the most decorated British Paralympian in history and a friend of mine. And then there was me, a mother of three, an amateur runner, captured in a quiet moment of extraordinary duality: athlete and mother, side by side. Standing there, it hit me. This wasn't just a running photo. It had flipped the male lens in sport to show something bigger. It represented a new way of seeing women.

Bolstered by the exhibition, I launched a survey to gather the opinions of thousands of female runners. I wanted to understand their barriers to entering races and the changes they wanted to see implemented. I knew the barriers I had faced, but I also knew we were all different. I officially set up SheRACES in June 2022, using the survey results as its launch pad, and, work-ing with several race directors, I used the findings to create a set of practical guidelines. It was a small non-profit Community Interest Company – initially with just me and some volunteers – with a mission to break down the barriers that prevent women from racing. The guidelines were the starting point and made it very simple to implement meaningful change at little cost, whether it was a 5k road race or a multi-day ultramarathon. The aim was never about simply changing pregnancy deferrals – it was about creating a better and more inclusive race experience overall: to get more women on the start line, to give them a better experience, and to equally value their competition. I'd paid for the start-up costs – building a website, branding, IT and more – with the money I'd received from two pieces of filming, one for Adidas Terrex and one for Emporio Armani on motherhood. All my time was volunteered, as it still is today. But I had no budget left for public relations. Luckily, I knew all the major journalists and magazines in the running world – I'd been interviewed enough times by them on my UTMB story – so I managed to secure initial coverage and it snowballed from there.

The months whizzed by and races started implementing the SheRACES guidelines, and I kept on training. Before I knew it, it was mid-September and I was five days out from running in the 24 Hour European Championships. I'd kept the whole race quiet, barely mentioning it to anyone and only posting on Instagram at the very last minute. Deep down, despite all the training, I still felt like I didn't belong. But the moment the Team GB kit landed on my doorstep, I couldn't help but feel a rush of excitement. Pulling out the blue, white and red striped vest with 'Great Britain' emblazoned across the chest was proof that I was officially representing my country.

But that buzz quickly turned to bemusement. The kit was exactly the same for every athlete, whether you were running 100 metres, throwing a discus or running for 24 hours. It was sleek, tight, and about as far from practical as you could get. The fabric screamed speed, not comfort. There were no seams designed with chafing in mind, no thought for what happens when your body is moving for a full day and night. Every athlete – no matter the distance or event – got the same choice of kit. With only one vest and one pair of shorts supplied there was no throwing up or soiling yourself, two unfortunate but common side effects of ultrarunning. I knew immediately I couldn't run in any of the short options. I needed my EVB support shorts for pelvic floor protection. Thankfully, with a bit of last-minute scrambling, I managed to get clearance to wear them, which was a weight off my mind.

The week before the race was absolute chaos. I wasn't just preparing for a championship; I was preparing my entire house-hold to run without me. The mental load was off the scale. I labelled every school and sports bag, created a spreadsheet mapping who needed to be where and when, laid out outfits for each day and had friends on standby for emergency pickups. I was packing for myself, for three kids, for their routines and somehow still supposed to be prioritising rest.

The period up to this moment had been anything but easy. I'd been through two kids starting new schools, caring for my mum who had just had an operation, juggling SheRACES projects and trying to be in peak physical condition to compete internationally. It was too much. Trying to calm my racing mind I visualised myself in the magnificent city of Verona, made famous by William Shakespeare's *Romeo and Juliet*. The romantic vision saw me flying through the charming streets of antiquity, representing my country while my teammates cheered me on. The dream was washed away the moment I stepped off the plane in Italy, replaced by the stark reality of industrial backstreets, strained smiles and the sinking feeling that I was an outsider.

Arriving in Verona I struggled to relax. I felt overwhelmed by the number of 24-hour athletes, many of whom had competed several times before and knew what to expect. I'd been selected to run as an individual, outside the official team of six. I was there to gain experience for future championships. Mealtimes were intense: two full women's and men's teams and solo runners like me meant a total of 16 athletes, plus crew, were all packed around large tables. I felt like I was constantly trying to find a corner to breathe. I also felt a complete fraud, like I'd slipped into someone else's kit by mistake.

Naively, I'd pictured the Verona course as a 1.6km loop through historic streets and grand squares. Instead, it wound around the back of industrial buildings, behind a row of smelly restaurants and overflowing bins. A few cracked pavements, the hum of delivery vans and a constant waft of fried food was not exactly the fairytale setting I'd imagined. The championships were supposed to be a celebration – my first GB vest, months of hard work and a step up on to the international stage – but in reality it was one of the hardest, most disappointing race experiences of my life. I'd barely made it to the start line in one piece, let alone in the mental space to switch off and focus. I felt trapped in my own head the whole way around.

From the outset the race seemed to be besieged with problems. My chip didn't work properly, and for hours I thought I was two miles down. It undermined my motivation, slowing me down and making me feel sad. It wasn't until after the race that Robbie kindly lobbied to have my true distance recorded with the use of Strava segments. Stomach issues also plagued me early on. I spent far too much time in the Portaloos, making 16 trips up and down a slope to reach them. Doubled over with gas cramps, I wasted a lot of time trying to settle my bowels.

Sports physiologist Dr Jamie Pugh, from Liverpool John Moores University, was my key crew member. While Jamie was a brilliant sports scientist with a wealth of experience, he wasn't John. We'd just met and I didn't know yet how to brief him properly about how to support me. It made me realise I worked best when crewed by John or a female crew member. Many delicate issues occur during ultrarunning and expressing them to a man you barely know is extremely uncomfortable (I've become a lot better at this since then). A stranger also doesn't know what mental buttons to push and when to put their foot down. That became painfully obvious when I started overheating. It was too hot and I refused an ice bandana – something John would never have allowed. I also didn't switch from my t-shirt to a vest in the morning, which was a big mistake. I ended up managing multiple things myself when all I wanted to do was zone out.

I was constantly thinking about my fuelling, my music and charging devices. As a result, my pacing began to unravel in the second half of the race. For the first 12 hours I had been on point, sticking to my pacing plan. My energy was high, despite the tummy troubles. I had managed to shift my period to its optimal point in my cycle, which was a huge help. I prefer to race between days six and 10 of my cycle when my fuelling requirements are lower. A limiter on my running is often how much food I can take in, so competing early in my cycle helps me fuel more efficiently. I really struggle racing in the last two weeks of my cycle, as I need to take in more fuel for the same performance than earlier in my cycle. A 24-hour race relies upon how much I can eat and drink, so if I can eat less to achieve the same performance, it's a massive advantage. I shift my cycle using simple progesterone pills. I start taking the pills a few days before my period is due, and then stop taking them two days before I want my period to come. I like to race just after it finishes. It's not that I can't race while on my period – I often feel strongest during it – but it's an added logistical burden in a 24-hour race, because of the impact on fuelling and having to worry about changing sanitary products.

Having moved my period for the race, I was able to run strong in the first half, fuelling well. But the second half was a different story. My neck collapsed, unable to bear the weight of exertion. I'd had issues before and hadn't fully resolved them. Videos showed my chin pointing to the sky, my posture all over the place. I could keep running, but it was wildly inefficient.

I relied on internal motivation, both positive and negative, to keep going. The carrot was the vision of finishing strong, the kids' excitement when I returned home, the pride in showing them what's possible. And the stick was how I would feel if I didn't finish or achieve my best performance. How would I tell the kids I hadn't tried my best? As always, I was assessing which voice cut through in the moment, using whichever one would move my feet forward. In those final few hours I felt gloomy and alone, but nothing was going to stop me from finishing. I might not finish strong, but I would be going home with a finish.

In the end, once my results were ratified, I ran a PB of 218.8km, finishing fourth out of seven in the women's team. I was gutted. On paper the result sounded good, but I knew it wasn't my best performance. Looking back on the photos my usual cheery demeanour was completely missing. I wasn't smiling in any of the pictures. I wasn't even present. I had not enjoyed the whole experience. No one judged me more critically than myself. Leaving Verona I felt deflated, but resolved to learn from the experience. I was only two years postpartum, and I was still very green in the world of 24-hour racing. That experience taught me what I needed to change next time. Because there would be a next time. I was sure of that. I no longer wanted to feel like an imposter. I was determined to prove the legitimacy of my place on the team.

Six months later and I was ready. Standing on the bright white starting line of Crawley racetrack I finally felt prepared. This was my chance to earn a spot at the 24 Hour World Championships in Taiwan in December 2023. The weather was kind, with no sign of April showers. Instead, it was a mild spring day and perfect conditions for racing. I knew I needed a much better distance than I'd run in Verona if I was going to make the GB team. The qualification standards had increased and I couldn't leave it to chance. I'd been building towards this for months – physically, mentally and logistically – and this race felt like my last shot.

By this point, John was no longer a novice at crewing. In fact, he'd become so confident he was managing other people's crews, coaching them through fuelling strategies and pacing advice. It was brilliant to watch him step into that role, but what meant most to me was how invested he was in my outcome. He wasn't just supporting anymore, he was pushing. He knew what I was capable of and made sure I didn't ease off at the end. It was also the first time I'd really lined up against others who were directly competing for GB places. There were five women with better PBs than me on the start list, all aiming for the remaining spots (some women had already run strong qualifiers). But I made a conscious decision to focus only on what I could control. I wasn't going to be drawn into racing anyone else. I broke the race into eight blocks of three hours, which helped give it structure. I approached it with calm and clarity. Paul Magee, a sports therapist who supported GB and Northern Ireland, was there crewing Ali Young (a previous GB representative) and had helped me ahead of the race, particularly with my neck, which had been causing me problems since Verona. He gave me gentle reminders to stretch and stay aligned – little nudges that really made a difference over 24 hours.

I'd meticulously planned my pacing and felt confident enough to stick to my plan. I reckoned 230km would get that spot. No need to go out fast like I did a year earlier at Walton-on-Thames. Keep it steady. When one of the other women racing for a GB spot went off hard and pulled ahead early on, I didn't panic. There were still so many hours left. I had to keep focused on my own goal, even as those around me chased national records and GB qualifiers. This was far more serious than my previous experience, with not a speck of fancy dress in sight. It was an IAU-licensed event (International Association of Ultrarunners) refereed by legendary GB ultrarunner Hilary Walker. As we coursed around the track I tuned into the world around me. I preferred to settle into my pace without music, using external distractions to keep my mind occupied, and save music for when I needed to go inside my head. I tuned into a football match on a nearby pitch, trying to guess which team had scored based on the size of the cheering. Mental strength is as important as physical in these races. I don't work formally with a sports psychologist, but luckily for me one of my running friends, Wendy Eason, is a brilliant one. Before each race I make sure to meet up for a run to talk through my strategies, focusing on finding my exact 'why' for that event and how I will stay in the moment when I feel overwhelmed. I draw on all of the challenges I have overcome in life – not just running – to give me strength. Much of it is through motherhood, whether that is dealing with sleep deprivation, or hearing the endless repetition of 'mummy mummy mummy' – great mental preparation for running in circles.

The first eight hours passed by without incident. My stomach was happy, my mood was high and food was going down easily. I'd discovered jam sandwiches (crusts off) were a superfood, lining my stomach to stop me feeling hungry, alongside jelly babies, gels, chews and bananas. As we entered the early evening, I switched to listening to light music, singing along in my head to a 2000s road trip playlist. I kept moving strongly through the early hours of the morning and shifted to internal distractions, something I could only maintain for a few hours. Going deep within myself, I visualised telling my 14-year-old self that this was her future. That she was capable of far more than she realised. I wished I could shout across the decades and wipe out those years of feeling my body wasn't good enough. That I was not an athlete. And before I knew it, I was entering the next day.

I love sunrise in a track race – the transition from the dark hours to seeing that first chink of light. Every lap the sun would visibly rise upwards, lighting up the sky with a mesmeric glow. I was feeling strong – better than any track race before. Everything had aligned. I just kept running and running. The only time I walked was a few metres to the toilets, half a dozen times in 24 hours. My focus was razor sharp with just one lapse in concentration when John disappeared for a quick nap in the car. He hadn't left any fuel prepped and I had to rummage around our kit trying to find a caffeine gel. It snapped me out of the rhythm briefly, but I got back on track quickly. I crossed the line having run 235.7km – my best ever performance, which placed me in the top 10 fastest British women of all-time, narrowly behind Hilary Walker herself (though she never had a pair of carbon shoes). I felt vindicated. I had done it. I had proved myself. The GB team selection was the following week, but I already knew it was mine. As we walked away from the track, clasping my glass trophy for first female, John told me, 'You've run further than you – or I – thought you could.' The kids weren't so impressed. Glass doesn't travel well to school for show-and-tell – they wouldn't be allowed to take it. But at least we had remembered to get a babysitter this time. As my parents scuttled out the door, our babysitter appeared, shooing John and I off to bed.

April was a month of mixed emotions. Team GB announced my selection for the World Championships along with three other women. But the men's team had six members. In these events, the three best performances per team are collated to create the overall team score. This meant there was huge pressure on the women's team, as only one person could underperform or drop out. Meanwhile, only half the men had to perform well (they had a stronger male contingency, so had decided to take a larger male team – not enough women qualified that year). I was angry at the disparity and the injustice of the selection, but there was nothing I could do. I was also conflicted over some SheRACES news. After years of our campaigning, UTMB had finally agreed to allow pregnant women to defer for five years. This was an amazing breakthrough, but the organisation was refusing to make a public announcement – so I had to take to social media once more to spread the word.

I was thrilled about the World Championships selection, but as usual I was being pulled in lots of different directions. I needed to get a handle on what to focus on, and how to train as effectively as possible. As a numbers person I decided to turn to the data. Listening to my body wasn't enough, because it was giving me false positives. The Crawley race had been a huge load on my body, the hardest I'd ever run. Ten days after the race I'd felt fine, but my resting heart rate was still high. This continued for the next four weeks and my appetite was insatiable. I was eating everything in sight, snacking on several slices of Nutella on toast a day between hearty meals. My heart rate variability also remained high (an indication that my nervous system was not back to normal). I became so concerned I messaged a friend at Garmin. I thought something was wrong with my watch. 'You're still recovering,' they assured me. Days later I received a message from Camille Herron, one of the best road ultrarunners in the world. She explained that her recovery took six to eight weeks after a similar effort, and I just needed to listen to the numbers. This was a turning point in understanding my body. I felt like I could have pushed hard again, but it would have delayed my recovery. The numbers were telling me to take it slow for a little while longer.

Thankfully I didn't have to wait too long. The summer months brought a new training block as I gradually increased running volume and intensity. It was another busy period juggling school holidays, running and everything SheRACES threw at me. In July I had a change of scenery attending the Active Pregnancy Awards, where I picked up gongs for Woman of the Year and Mother Athlete of the Year. It felt brilliant to bring the two sides of my life together – performance and advocacy – and celebrate with an amazing group of women in sport. A few days later I managed to fit in a last-minute escape to Eiger Ultra Trail in Switzerland with Matt. After failing to buy a place from another competitor (a common practice on Facebook), for the first time ever I had sneakily leaned into my Instagram following and the profile I had from SheRACES. I asked the race organisers for a place in return for giving them feedback on the accessibility of the race to women. Luckily, they said yes. It was a boiling hot day, but I made it through the beautiful 101km course thanks to carrying two litres of water, rather than the mandatory one litre, after I analysed the checkpoint gaps. For every race, especially in the mountains or on technical terrain, I analyse the checkpoint splits of past competitors similar to my pace, so I know how long I'll likely take between water stops. On the flight home I ate most of the Swiss chocolates I'd bought for the kids and quickly picked up some Percy Pigs at M&S to replace them.

Training, campaigning and family days out became my daily routine. Eddie was happy with my progress, and everything seemed to be going to plan when suddenly a huge spanner was thrown in the works. I was in my peak training period, honing in on endurance and speed, ensuring nothing disrupted my sessions. On the Tom Evans spectrum (the scale I had invented following my successful UTMB finish) I was at 80 per cent, the maximum I was willing to go to. Then six weeks before the World Championships in Taiwan John had a horrific cycling accident. We had managed to organise three days away together on a cycling retreat in Ibiza – just the two of us. While I couldn't risk cycling in a group so close to the world champs, I was happy to run and cycle solo while John joined group rides. There had been a couple of hairy moments for John on the first day where he had to take evasive action, so he was more nervous than usual about riding in a peloton.

On day two we planned to meet for lunch following his morning ride. I'd run early then cycled to the group lunch meeting point, where we had a breathwork session. I didn't know how quickly I'd be needing those breathing techniques. Suddenly my phone rang. I had a sinking feeling in the pit of my stomach. Was this how John felt when I collapsed in Cambodia? A voice at the end of the line told me to come quick. John had crashed after the bike in front had braked suddenly with no warning. Swerving to avoid it, he was thrown off his own bike, breaking both his ankle and elbow. Panic stations. I reached him just after the ambulance arrived. I could barely look. His face was haunted by pain, his rosy cheeks bleached to an ashen grey. He tried to tell me he was OK, always thinking of me, but I knew it was serious. Moments later he was driven away to the local hospital, and I headed straight back to the hotel to pack our gear. We needed to leave immediately. That evening we flew straight home and John was transferred to hospital for emergency surgery.

It was my turn to look after John. I considered myself a physically strong woman, but having a husband with a broken ankle and elbow (on the same side) brought considerable challenges. His elbow was permanently damaged and until this day he still can't fully straighten it. Having a break in both sets of limbs meant using crutches was out of the question. The first dilemma was how to get John into the house. Our entrance is up a series of steps and I wasn't strong enough to carry him. He ended up crawling his way through the front door before I helped him on to one foot. He was completely immobile and totally reliant on me.

The situation felt so unfair. I could train and he couldn't. I was preparing for the World Championships, and he would never be able to play his beloved racket sports to the same standard with the kids again. The strain of looking after him and the kids became immense, but he was my number-one concern, and in that moment running seemed frivolous. I even wondered if I should, or could, actually go to Taiwan. I managed almost all of the training Eddie set, but family sacrifices had to be made to do that. Donnacha and Saoirse missed out on big birthday parties as I couldn't manage the planning, having a sleepover and family tea instead (which in hindsight they enjoyed just as much). Homemade birthday cake was replaced with shop bought and I leaned heavily on local friends to help. It couldn't have come at a worse time, but even more difficult was seeing John struggle.

We agreed as a family that Taiwan was too big an opportunity to miss, but I felt awful prioritising my training. And it wasn't just about getting race fit – I also needed to climatise. Taiwan would be hot, humid and polluted, and I needed a strategy to cope in the heat. Installing an infrared sauna in the garage – a birthday present from John earlier in the year (a particularly extravagant present, because I hadn't asked for a birthday gift for several years) – enabled me to heat train and get used to my core body temperature rising. I was in shape to run 240+km, but I knew the climate would slow me down. I had to calculate a realistic reduction in pace. With only four of us in the team, I couldn't risk going out too fast and then having to pull out. I settled on pacing for 225km.

My experience from Crawley had taught me how to manage a 24-hour race, but I also needed to make changes to my pre-race routine. I knew being around other people – and too much testosterone – overstimulated me and I needed a calmer lead-in. Longing for peace and low energy, I decided to remove myself from the group when we arrived in sticky Taiwan a few days before the race. I shared a room with just one other person – Sarah Cameron – who had been selected by the head of the GB team to crew me. My feedback had been listened to following Verona, and they recognised I needed a female crew member this time. It was quiet, calm and gave me the headspace I needed and a lot of time with Sarah to talk about my strategy.

The day before the race, I wandered off alone to the National Museum of Taiwan, escaping the growing buzz of the event. My mum had been recovering from another operation and she loved ceramics, so I took videos of painted pots and vases, sending them back to her with voice notes about their origins. It felt grounding; a reminder that there was a world outside the loop I was about to run. Another connection to home came in the unexpected form of a jam sandwich. I stumbled across a little supermarket and found, to my delight, shelves stocked with ready-made jam sandwiches – sealed at the edges, crusts already cut off and available in all sorts of flavours. I raided three stores then asked the crew to buy every single one they could find on their bigger supermarket trip.

One of the highlights of that week was catching up with American runner Camille Herron in person for the first time. Eszter Csillag, another elite ultrarunner, joined too, in Taiwan to crew for the New Zealand team. I worked closely with Eszter on the Pro Trail Runners Women's Committee, supporting elite athletes in trail running. The three of us stood talking for what felt like hours, putting the world to rights. Despite being in the company of women I once considered unreachable, it felt natural. That sense of belonging carried into the opening ceremony, when I was asked to carry the flag for Team GB. It was an honour and, in true Sophie fashion, a bit of a chaotic one. The flag kept whipping about, flailing in all directions as I tried to walk with poise. The rest of the team laughed kindly, teasing me about my wild flag-waving technique. But this time, unlike Verona, I didn't feel out of place. I felt accepted.

Race day arrived and we looked the part, kitted out in ice vests like seasoned pros. The course was a 2km loop, including a gauntlet of crew tables where each team had their designated pit stop. The streets were closed for the 300 runners, which included 110 women. Lining up, sweat already dripping off me in the 80 per cent humidity, felt surreal. This wasn't just a run. It was the culmination of years of work, fluctuating goals and seeking purpose. We set off at 10 a.m., some racing ahead, others like me sticking to a more conservative pace. For 24 hours I looped through the city, past lantern-lit stalls and kids riding bikes. The route went through a bustling city park in Taipei, winding past fountains, trees and stretches of concrete path. Every lap took us past a giant red hotel with an ornamental roof, a surreal anchor point in the otherwise repetitive course. In the early stages, the hotel was a bustling hive of activity, visitors coming and going. As the race wore on, I watched it change. The lights dimmed, the curtains closed, the lobby emptied out. Nearby a café bar with easy afternoon vibes transformed into a nightclub, playing a different song each time I ran past, calling me to join the party. Taipei's culture unfolded before my eyes and I felt privileged to experience this slice of 24 hours in the city.

As expected, the conditions were hot, in the mid-20s, with air pollution making it more difficult to breathe. At the halfway mark I was sitting in 40th place out of 111 women. But I knew my strength lay in the second half. As the night progressed, I moved steadily through the field. Unfortunately, my teammates weren't doing so well. They began dropping one by one, leaving me the only British woman on the course. Once the second woman was out, we lost all hope of a team medal. I couldn't help but feel a pang of jealousy watching the men's team, who had strong support and camaraderie. My race became a solo one and with that a feeling of isolation crept in. By 2 a.m. I'd started to overheat and was struggling to stay cool. The crew were in puffer jackets while I was pouring cold water over my head. I was start-ing to crack and was in desperate need of a rest. The crew's job was to keep runners out of the tent, to keep them moving, but they took one look at me and let me crash. They knew I didn't stop when I didn't need to. We had no shot at a team medal and I wasn't in contention for a solo one, so it seemed reasonable to allow me to nap. At 3 a.m. I took a five-minute sleep break in a tent behind the British crew table, just enough to reset physi-cally and mentally, before I was quickly ushered outside.

The final hours felt immensely lonely. The other members of the women's team had gone back to the hotel and the crew team were rightly focused on ensuring the men secured their bronze medal. Women and men weren't allowed to run together, so even though I was lapping at the same pace as some male teammates I was not allowed to tag on. My dream of racing in a team had been crushed, but I didn't feel dispirited. I was racing for my country on the world stage. Me, the chubby 14-year-old girl who came second to last in the school mile, was competing in the same vest as some of my athletic heroines. It was beyond my wildest dreams. I belonged on the track and finally had the self-belief that I deserved to be there. I had picked off 92 runners in the field and finished in 19th place. I was the first British woman, having paced it exactly right. With that result my imposter syndrome finally lifted. I might not look like a typical endurance athlete with my stocky build and muscly arms, but one thing was undeniable. I was very good at running very long distances. And I had finally been accepted.

The next morning we went for a team hike up a mountain to keep our muscles moving, and for the crew to laugh at how some of us couldn't go down the stairs that wound around the mountain. I was surprised at how good I felt; not as exhausted as I was after Crawley. I then caught an Uber into the city for the mandatory buying of presents for the kids, but also to walk around, getting a feel for the different districts and embracing the opportunity to be in a new country.

I had been hoping to find some Beyblade toys, which were my eldest son's latest obsession, but after traipsing through multiple department stores realised they were Korean rather than Taiwanese and they weren't a 'thing' here yet. Fortunately, I found a Pokemon version, where a Pikachu spinner popped out of a Pokeball, which I knew would thrill the kids, as would the random selection of sweets I amassed from the local supermarket.

That night I went out to celebrate with the men's team and the rest of the GB crew at the local night market. Finally I was able to try all the different dishes on offer – things that would have been far too risky stomach-wise before the race. I bought everything that called out to me, my body desperate to get calories in, with second helpings of deep-fried ice cream with chocolate sauce.

After a 14-hour flight home, where I got a luxurious sleep spread across a row of four seats after my teammates upgraded theirs, I arrived back home. Donnacha, Cormac and Saoirse met me with the biggest cuddles possible. 'Mummy, you're amazing,' they said. 'We saw you on the TV! Were you really the best runner in the whole of Britain?' And then, of course, 'Did you bring home any sweets?' And in that moment, there was no better finish line.

Coda: You belong

After years of juggling babies, recovery and racing windows, I finally had the space to chase performance and not just finish lines. With our family complete, I felt physically strong again, mentally ready and deeply motivated. I found myself stronger than ever at the Maverick South Downs race and a fire was lit. I set my sights on Spartathlon, wanting not just to finish but to truly perform. And then I got the shock of my life: a place on the GB team. I didn't feel like I belonged. Me, the girl who came second last in the school mile. But standing in my GB kit, despite the chaos of training, mum duties and imposter syndrome, I realised I *had* arrived. After years of pregnancy, prolapse and postpartum, I had finally made it: from pregnancy to performance. I could stand tall amongst my idols and believe that I was, indeed, a world-class runner.

11

CHALLENGE YOURSELF

Ireland–Crossing World Record

Salty tears streamed down my face. I was bawling like a baby, face screwed up into an ugly, snivelly mess. Each sob shook my exhausted body as I strode forward along the endless country road. I had been running on tarmac for 56 hours, in the driving Irish rain. My swollen left knee poked painfully through a swathe of pink strapping, an orange support earnestly holding it in place. My face was fixed into a permanent grimace, afraid to relax, holding my body and resolve firm. The tears stung my raw, weathered cheeks as they rolled ungraciously into the unrelenting wind – not tears of pain or defeat, but of overwhelming emotion as a dream became reality. Ahead of me a chorus of excited voices grew louder, the initial hum transforming into a sea of animated screams.

The wall of beaming faces had spent the morning painstakingly crafting personalised messages of support. Now they stood proudly outside their school, signs aloft as they chanted my name. The enthusiasm was infectious and, despite the weight of my weariness, I suddenly felt a surge of uplifting energy. As I glanced back, a line of children dressed in red and navy-blue PE kits filed in behind me. My tears grew bigger, clouding my vision. Girls with long plaited hair, bright-eyed with admiration, shouted words that pierced my heart: 'We want to be like you, Sophie!' It was this genuine outpouring from these Irish schoolchildren that finally broke me, filling my soul with a sense of purpose, reminding me why I had undertaken this incredible challenge. In that emotionally charged moment the journey became so much more significant than the result. I was attempting my first world record, but more importantly I was demonstrating to those hopeful girls just what was possible.

From the outset my mantra had been 'one woman, one girl'. If I could get just one female to view themselves differently because of my run, then it would all be worth it. I was only running for three days. It was nothing in a lifetime. But if I could impact someone's life, and how they saw themselves and their potential, then they would have that for the rest of their life. No matter how much I hurt this was a really good use of three days of my life. In that moment, as I ran past Caherline National School in Limerick, I realised it was no longer one girl, it was dozens. The tears kept pouring.

The true genesis of this highly personal quest had emerged thousands of miles away, months earlier, in the humid air of Taiwan. At the World Championships in December 2023 I'd realised something powerful about myself: I thrived over longer distances. After 12 hours of running, I'd been in 40th place, but by the end of a full day I had finished 19th in the world, gradually moving my way through the field. I felt like I had more to give. My energy was not depleted. This realisation made me aware of a resilience I hadn't fully acknowledged before and a quiet confidence began to stir inside me. On the flight back to Europe, sitting alongside the Irish running team, a seed was planted during casual conversations about running records, specifically the challenge of running the length of Ireland from Malin to Mizen Head – a distance of 558km. Ed McGroarty, a member of the Irish team, had the men's record and the idea instantly connected with me. I had travelled to Taiwan alone, leaving my family and a host of childcare complexities behind me. I'd really wanted them by my side to witness and celebrate my best performance to date, but it was just too far. I longed for an adventure we could share together. And it just so happened that my husband was from Ireland.

The notion took root deep within my imagination, bursting through the surface during a transformative moment at the Running Industry Alliance conference shortly after my return from Taiwan. As I sat in the audience, still recovering from the championship race, elite trail runner Ellis Bland unexpectedly pointed to my recent achievements, encouraging questions from the crowd about long-distance endurance. For the first time I felt seen; recognised as an athlete worthy of admiration and respect from those I saw as elites. I was just a mother of three and had never viewed myself as an elite contender. I had always felt fraudulent, an imposter alongside the 'proper' athletes. This validation propelled my thoughts further: perhaps I could undertake something monumental, not just for personal achievement but to inspire a broader community, particularly women. Perhaps I wasn't so bad at this long-distance malarky after all. Perhaps I was capable of breaking a world record.

Still riding high from my success in Taiwan it didn't take long for the pieces to fall into place. My calendar was clear and I had space for a long recovery. The next 24 Hour World Championships were more than a year away, and we had nothing planned for the May half-term school holiday in 2024 – so I thought this would be an opportune week to slot in a world record attempt. The more I thought about it, the more the Irish quest made sense. I wanted a challenge that was more than 24 hours long, that could heavily involve my family and that would impact people at a grassroots level. SheRACES was making inroads with race organisers, and a growing number were changing their policies and signing up to the guidelines. But there was still a massive gap in female participation in ultras. Start lines were often made up of 80 per cent or more men, and they remained a space where many women felt they didn't belong. Wanting to encourage more women to sign up for races I was eager to create a huge symbolic gesture that screamed 'women can do tough stuff!' By pushing myself to the limit I could provoke others into action and normalise going outside your comfort zone.

My previous experience of the Summer Spine Race – 431km over five days – had given me insight into the balance between running at pace and getting very little sleep. I understood how tiredness affected me and felt I could use lack of sleep to my advantage. Mimi Anderson was the current Guinness World Record Holder of the fastest crossing of Ireland on foot by a female. In 2012 she set a phenomenal record of 87 hours 36 minutes and 55 seconds. Mimi was an idol of mine, having set countless course and world records, including running 1352km from John O'Groats to Land's End in 12 days and becoming the first woman to complete a double Comrades ultramarathon in South Africa covering 176km (running Comrades twice in one continuous go). Her record would be incredibly difficult to beat. She had set off from Malin Head in the north of Ireland at an outstanding pace, running the first marathon in three hours and 36 minutes. By the time she'd reached the southerly finish point at Mizen Head, Mimi had knocked a colossal 10 hours off the previous record.

The only way I felt I could beat her time would be to cut back on sleep and stops. While Mimi had the luxury of sleeping in the back of a van – she slept for a total of 4.5 hours during the crossing – I planned to power nap by the roadside. Sleep, or a lack of it, was a major part of my strategy, along with a strict caffeine regime – for which I'd built a detailed Excel model to tell me how much I could take without detrimental effects on my gut. The distance was not the only appeal of Ireland. It was deeply personal. My husband was from County Cork and we'd given all our children Irish names, but the kids rarely spent time in the country, only popping over for short visits to see grandparents, aunts and cousins. I thought it would be an amazing experience for the boys, then aged six and nine, to travel the whole country with me. Meanwhile, three-year-old Saoirse, who was too young to enjoy the travelling, would be waiting for me at my in-laws west of Cork. The image etched into my mind was clear and powerful: running as fast as physically possible back home to my daughter waiting for me at granny and grandad's house. That vision became my constant companion, a beacon through exhaustion, injury and torrential rain. Each step wasn't simply a stride closer to a record; it was a heartbeat closer to her.

Running home to Saoirse represented something even more profound than personal ambition. It symbolised my wider mission – to inspire and empower other women. From my work as a trustee of Women in Sport I was acutely aware of the limits girls placed on themselves from as young as five. Girls don't think they are as good as boys at sport and this negatively manifests as women become older. Women have five hours less leisure time than men per week and find it difficult to prioritise their own wellbeing. Here was my opportunity to set a powerful example, and challenge other women and girls to test their physical boundaries. It could be running to the nearest town or cycling to work for the first time. It could be anything meaningful and uncomfortable. I decided to name the attempt 'Challenge You' to inspire other women to take on their own challenges. I now had three compelling reasons to attempt the world record. To push myself further than before, to connect with my children's Irish heritage and to inspire other women. There was nothing left to consider. I was going to Ireland.

In these types of extreme challenges the athlete is only as good as their crew. I needed to assemble a strong group of people around me to help manage childcare, logistics and keeping me fuelled. Quite by chance I had met the record-breaking cyclist Kate Strong at the Running Industry Alliance conference in December 2023. We connected momentarily as I was rushing home and joked that with the names Power and Strong we had to be friends, so we exchanged numbers and promised to chat further. On a call a few weeks later I told Kate about my desire to take on the Ireland record. In the next breath Kate declared she was coming to cycle alongside me. I was shocked. I didn't know this woman. We hadn't even met properly and she was willing to give up a week of her life to cycle non-stop across another country. As a world record endurance cyclist, she sensed I might be able to break the record and didn't want to miss out. Her belief in me was incredibly powerful and I immediately knew I wanted her by my side.

A former aerospace engineer, I realised she would be great at problem-solving – and it proved to be true. Once in Ireland Kate took control of the crew as she meticulously logged my hydration, food and kit. She ensured I was taking the right amount of salts, snacks and caffeine gels starting at 10 p.m. each night. Her spreadsheet had 20 columns ensuring I had warm gloves at exactly the right moment, a top-up of suntan lotion before I started to burn and that my temperature was checked every evening. She also reminded me to reapply chafing cream to avoid rubbing as much as possible. With three Guinness World Records to her name, Kate understood how to dot the i's and cross the t's to ensure Guinness had all the evidence they needed. And the list was long. I needed a professional GPS tracking device, visible to all online so people could join me, my GPS running watch recording cadence (showing I was running and not in a car!) and as many independent witnesses as possible (not family or friends) to sign a logbook along the way, a task often given to Donnacha and Cormac so they could be involved.

Every time I stopped for any reason this had to be logged and a photo with a clock time had to be taken. There was no dashing into the bushes for anything more than a quick wee, the stop had to be logged, explained and photographed first. Then there was the issue of video footage, which had to include the start and finish, notable landmarks on the route and at least 10 minutes of film every 24 hours. While I was concentrating on keeping ahead of Mimi's tough record my crew would be running around detailing the route in a spreadsheet, taking photos, and keeping hold of receipts of every Red Bull, ice cream or cup of tea purchased for me as I ran.

With Christmas out of the way I met face to face with Kate in early 2024 and we started planning in earnest. I wanted the children to be involved in the record attempt, but since Donnacha and Cormac were in school the best window of opportunity was still May half-term. I would have enough time to train and put logistics in place, but on the downside I would have to run whatever the weather – there was no wriggle room given that the school break was only one week. Childcare was nonetheless a dilemma, and my first call was to my in-laws in Ireland. They had booked a holiday that week, but were about to cancel as they had yet another grandchild on the way. This meant they were able to look after Saoirse, while John drove the rented motorhome, taking Donnacha and Cormac to every recreational football pitch along the route so they could let off steam.

Kate was there to cycle behind me, keeping me safe on the roads. I also enlisted my dear friend Nick, the founder of Impact Marathon, and his new wife Liza Ponce who took over my social media as volunteer crew. Nick had sold the week to her as a lovely road trip across Ireland. Liza had no idea what she was in for. Later she told me that being cooped up in a van, having no sleep for three nights and working together under pressure was the best relationship test they could have. They were now more prepared than ever to start a family together. Nick and Liza's job was to staff the smaller camper van following me as a food and bedding supply unit (while John was in the motorhome with the boys providing logistical support).

Capturing the photography and videography was Phil Hill tagging alongside Liza and Nick, who was tasked with documenting the run not only for Guinness, but for the wider public as part of the Challenge You initiative (which I self-funded). I had worked with Phil before, during my pregnancy when he made the film about my recovery jour-ney for Hoka, and knew he would be a great addition to the team. Phil created an incredible film of the challenge which later premiered at Kendal Film Festival during the Women in Adventure night. Seeing people brought to tears by the weight of my efforts was profoundly moving, a sign that the impact reached far beyond those I'd met on the road.

The pieces were falling into place. My training was going well, the crew were secured and my spreadsheet was starting to fill up. There was just one more person I needed to speak to: Mimi Anderson.

I had randomly met Mimi in my early ultrarunning days at a checkpoint toilet. She appeared to be running 50 miles on nothing more than a few jelly babies, and radiated positivity and joy. I had huge admiration for her. She had taken up running in her late thirties and gone on to win so many races, complete a double Spartathlon and many other amazing feats. Since I was gunning for her Ireland-crossing record, I felt it important to reach out to her. She showed me nothing but support. She embodied everything I loved about ultrarunning. Women were always supporting other women. None of us owned a record, we were simply looking after it for the next person. Mimi was incredibly generous with her time, and chatted to me about her crew and the logistics of the challenge. Throughout my attempt she was avidly watching my progress, sending me messages of support. It was more than a year later that Mimi admitted it had been incredibly tough to watch me break her record. 'I cried,' Mimi said. 'It was the last record I set before I had to stop running and it felt like it was all over for me. But equally I was so pleased for Sophie as she worked so hard for it. It was not my record. I was just the custodian.'

As I climbed into the passenger seat of the enormous six-berth motorhome, the reality of what lay ahead began to dawn on me. The nine-hour journey from Cork to the northern tip of Ireland – not even the full route I would run – seemed never-ending, the sheer length of the drive reinforcing the enormity of the impending challenge. Ireland was a big country. The length of it was a long way. I felt sick with anticipation.

The day hadn't got off to the best start. We had arrived on the Friday night, staying with John's family before doing a massive supermarket shop on Saturday. We stocked up on wraps, jam, avocado, bananas, crips, sweets, chocolate bars, hummus and more – enough to keep me fuelled on the move for three and a half days (as well as the crew). I was aiming for 300 calories an hour for as long as possible, topped up by chips and ice cream bought along the route, taking my total calorie intake to over 20,000. The plan was to eat twice an hour in the first couple of days, then at least once an hour when my pace slowed down.

Fuelling sorted, John went to collect the motorhome from a local rental company. The vehicle was ginormous. It could sleep six people and had plenty of room for all my food and spare clothes, plus space for the boys to hang out. This vehicle was going to be used to restock the smaller camper, driven by Nick and Liza. The motorhome was there as a back-up support vehicle and roomy enough for the boys to sleep in, but it was the camper that directly followed me down the small windy roads. In hindsight, the motorhome was perhaps a little too large. On Sunday morning as we were about to head north to the start of the run, while reversing out of his parent's drive John hit their gatepost, causing a massive scrape to the rear bumper. We hadn't even started the challenge and the vehicle was already pranged! This was additional stress we did not need. Fortunately, the damage was superficial and we were soon on our way.

Reaching Malin Head, the most northerly point of mainland Ireland, we regrouped with the rest of the team on Monday afternoon. They had taken the overnight ferry and were absolutely knackered. Having never crewed me before I needed to explain my expanse of kit to them. An explosion of clothing, food and accessories littered the inside of our Airbnb as I catalogued my gear to Kate, Nick and Liza.

We were also chasing Guinness witnesses as we needed two people – who were strangers to us – to witness the start of the record. Finally, we got word through a local Facebook group that two teachers would be showing up. All we could do was cross our fingers and toes in the hope they would turn up at 8 a.m. the next day. Otherwise I wouldn't be running anywhere.

That night I filled my tummy with fish and chips at the pub before trying to get an early night. It didn't feel like a good night's sleep, but when I woke up my Garmin told me I was in prime condition with a score of 100/100. If my watch thought I was ready, who was I to challenge it?

Standing at the rugged tip of Ireland, Malin Head stretched out before me, a beautifully wild landscape battered by relentless Atlantic winds. Jagged cliffs dropped sharply into the swirling sea below, where white-tipped breakers crashed endlessly against dark, unyielding rock. The air was thick with the tang of salt and sea spray, carried inland by gusts that bent the emerald green vegetation. The vast expanse of ocean stretching to the horizon was a dramatic reminder of the daunting task ahead of me.

I prepared to take my first steps, feeling the immense scale of my journey weighing heavily on my shoulders. And I felt the weight both physically and metaphorically, as the torrential rain lashed down on me. I ducked into a stone shelter, loaded up the route on my watch and hugged the boys tightly. John gently suggested delaying the start by a few hours, but my tight schedule left no room for flexibility. I was pacing for an 80-hour finish, meaning I could see my kids before bedtime on Friday. To break the record, I needed to reach Mizen Head before 11 p.m. that night and I didn't want my kids to be tired and grumpy. Better to get there late afternoon. If I stuck to my pacing strategy, I'd arrive around 4 p.m. and have plenty of time to see the kids. It was now or never; I couldn't delay my start. Determined, I pulled my hood tight around my face, took a deep breath and stepped out of the shelter into the relentless downpour, watched by two local witnesses. The time was officially 8 a.m. sharp.

Those initial solo miles were a mixture of exhilaration and apprehension. I deliberately chose to run alone at first, craving the headspace to mentally settle into the enormity of the challenge. The quiet solitude allowed me to focus on my rhythm, each step bringing me deeper into the lush landscapes of County Donegal. Despite the relentless rain, there was a beauty in those first few miles; the sound of my footsteps, the splashes through growing puddles and the stark, dramatic scenery provided an oddly calming backdrop. I was purposefully moving slower than

Mimi's pace, but I knew she had slowed significantly in the second half. I was making good progress and I reminded myself to stick to the plan. Up and down the country roads I went, through the pouring rain, constantly changing my waterproof jacket in a hopeless bid to remain dry.

As the miles ticked by and the landscape blurred, I found a surprising source of entertainment in the election posters adorning every lamppost and roadside fence. These massive faces and bold slogans marked my progress through each area, signalling new towns and shifting political allegiances. With little understanding of Irish politics, I amused myself by examining the curious choices each candidate made – stern expressions meant to convey seriousness, overly enthusiastic smiles attempting friendliness and slogans that ranged from the inspirational to the downright peculiar. These posters became a game, a cheerful distraction keeping my mind occupied along the long and arduous route.

Back at the camper van the crew were still finding their feet. Largely inexperienced but eager, they had the unenviable task of navigating country roads and learning on the job how to support an ultraendurance run. John was occupied with the boys, occasionally stopping off for impromptu football games or to gather witness statements, leaving Kate cycling beside me, juggling my immediate needs and safety. Her presence became a comforting constant, a steady anchor amidst the chaotic uncertainty of the road ahead. She cycled beside me for long stints, resting periodically in the van when other runners came out to join me.

Fuelling quickly emerged as a critical problem. Initially, I'd underestimated how frequently I needed sustenance, foolishly setting out with just a small waist belt containing minimal snacks and water. After a marathon distance into Londonderry, the first large town, I felt my energy reserves crashing dramatically. My crew were nowhere to be seen and Kate had disappeared in search of food. I'd been alone for over an hour without eating, each mile becoming more difficult as hunger gnawed at my stomach. Finally, Kate returned with some hastily acquired McDonald's chips, but without ketchup they were dry and unsatisfying. This was not going well. We needed a re-evaluation. The crew had no experience and John was tied up entertaining the boys, trying to advise the crew from afar. Everyone was doing the best they could, but it was far from perfect. We all realised how crucial constant, effective fuelling would be – this wasn't just about endurance, it was a battle against depletion – so Kate and the crew swiftly recalibrated, recognising the urgent need to drastically improve the nutritional strategy. From then on, my crew became vigilant about regular, calorie-dense intake, meticulously preparing jam tortilla wraps and bundles of sweets to help sustain me.

I tried my hardest to be kind to the team – they had given up so much for me – but I was not without my moments. At one point I refused a jam tortilla on the grounds that it did not have enough jam in it. I also lost my mind over a ham and cheese toasty on day two. I was craving the salty goodness and was adamant that the toastie must not contain mustard. I hated mustard. I couldn't have the tiniest bit. I'd been waiting for what seemed like hours for this holy grail of melted cheese and warm ham. I was so excited, salivating at the mere thought of it. Finally, it appeared. This was going to be worth the wait. Ugh! It had mustard in it. The crew swore blind that it didn't. I swore blind that it did. I was distraught. My amazing crew remained impeccably calm and patient – but they didn't offer me a toastie again!

As I approached the first night, I was feeling calm and focused. I had run on my own, passing a few well-wishers on the side of the road every so often. There were no crowds or people wanting to join me for a few miles. It was just what I wanted. My crew were learning how to handle me, cutting the tops of gels, opening packages for me and taking away all my rubbish. They asked about blisters, pointed out public toilets and told me how I was performing against Mimi's record. Around 2 a.m. I attempted to grab 20 minutes sleep in the van, but it was no use. All my 24-hour races meant my body was accustomed to running through the night and it was impossible to fall asleep. There was too much adrenaline coursing through my veins. I had to keep moving.

I set my sights on reaching Longford, the 209km marker glowing in my thoughts, where I knew Ciara would be waiting. Ciara and I had been close friends since I was 17 and over the years our bond had deepened – her son, Oisín, was now besties with Saoirse. Seeing Ciara wasn't just about friendly support; it was a comforting beacon guiding me through the night. I put some music on, Kate riding behind me in silence, and pushed on. The rain was pelting down at a 45-degree angle and I felt miserable. But there was nothing to do but keep on running. We were on the N87 through the night – a fast road where we clung to the hard shoulder and slurped caffeine gels to stay awake.

Before meeting Kate, I hadn't thought about having a cyclist. I just assumed it would be me running with occasional company and intermittent crew points. In this first night I realised how lucky I was to have her by my side, not just for logistical support and safety, but also for her hilarious tales of dating apps, which I summoned when I needed a laugh or two. At 4 a.m. we finally had relief as we turned on to a regional, quieter road. It led us out of Country Cavan, into County Leitrim and through 50km of farmland, on to our next goal.

By early morning the relentless rain had reduced to a persistent drizzle, coating everything in a glistening sheen. I finally reached Longford at 8.30 a.m., my spirits instantly lifting as I spotted Ciara waving energetically from the roadside. She'd printed out giant pictures of my face and plastered them boldly across the van, turning our crew vehicle into a cheerful mobile billboard. Seeing her familiar face and the playful images felt like a warm hug, reminding me how much I was loved and supported. Despite my best effects to eat through the early hours, nibbling wine gums and Precision Hydration chews, I was now really low on energy. An extra-large Cornetto and Red Bull from the garage were the breakfast pick-me-up that I needed.

The day brought with it a welcome wave of company as local ultrarunners began to join me. Brian Ahern from *The Runners Diary* podcast had spread the word and Stephen Murphy, who was soon to become Ireland's 100-mile record holder, appeared to pace me effortlessly for nearly 20km. Kate, who'd loyally cycled beside me since the start, finally got a much-needed break, handing me safely into Stephen's experienced care. We chatted easily about training strategies, the camaraderie feeling natural and reassuring. Just as Stephen departed, another ultra-runner Ed Payne smoothly took his place, continuing the relay of stories and encouragement that reminded me why I cherish the ultrarunning community.

At one point a peloton of 200 cyclists came careering towards me. They were crossing Ireland by bike in the opposite direction to me as part of a charity fundraiser. They were incredulous when they heard I was running the same route in a similar time. As the hours breezed by more and more runners appeared, eager to share miles and offer support. I was carrying a live tracker so anyone could see where I was at any given point in time. Liza took care of my social media channels, constantly updating my progress and adding photographs. Kate resumed her role as protector and guide, carefully instructing each newcomer with clear, assertive briefings about where to position themselves and how best to run alongside me. I was joined by many of the Sanctuary Runners, a unique running club who foster solidarity and friendship between Irish residents, migrants, asylum seekers and refugees. Among these supportive runners, there was one unfortunate exception – an energy-sapping presence who inserted himself beside me. He spoke little, providing no conversation or comfort, instead becoming a mental drain I simply couldn't afford. Feeling my energy ebb, I shot Kate a pleading glance, hoping she'd recognise my distress. Immediately catching on, she intervened swiftly and firmly, diplomatically saying I needed space. Relieved, I pressed forward, feeling profoundly grateful for her decisive action.

Kate continued to be a lifeline through the good, the bad and the damn right ugly. At first I was quite coy, hiding my modesty behind a bush when I went for a wee. Kate was having none of it. 'You don't have time to hide to pee. Just lean against me to save your quads.' Kate was right. She graciously knelt down – never complaining when my pee ended up spraying on her. I hardly knew her, but we were in this together.

During the second day, when things started to get very uncomfortable, Kate ensured I was 'ship shape and shining' down below. I'd started developing the most horrendous saddle sores on my bum. All that crouching in hedgerows to pee, barely able to clean up properly, combined with the constant wet weather and friction from running gear was a recipe for disaster. I could barely sit and even running became this strange negotiation with my own backside. Every time I moved, I winced. I knew exactly what I needed: the yellow tube; that magical, thick, soothing cream that had saved me during previous ultra events; the one specifically made for babies and nappy rash but which, in times like this, worked just as well for ultrarunners.

'I need the yellow tube!' I shouted to my crew between grimaces. Unfortunately, the crew thought I meant the yellow tube that lived in the van's kitchen supplies – the one filled with washing-up liquid. Thankfully, John, in the nick of time, realised exactly what I was talking about. He disappeared off to the nearest pharmacy returning with Metanium like a hero, holding that familiar yellow tube like it was a golden trophy. I could've cried with gratitude.

Then came the next challenge: applying it. By this point I was too sore to twist around or delicately dab it myself. I was done with shame. Everything was hurting, and I just needed help. I turned to Kate, a stranger who had become my closest ally, and said 'I need you to put this on me.' She didn't even flinch – she simply took the tube and got to work with calm, clinical efficiency. There we were, on the side of some backroad in Ireland, me bent awkwardly over while Kate carefully applied nappy rash cream to my most intimate body parts.

With one disaster averted there was soon another knocking aggressively at the door. Later the same day the crew realised we were in serious danger of running out of Precision Hydration gels. Two days of fruit-based gels and jelly babies had left my mouth sore and I now winced with anything acidic. It might not sound like a crisis, but for me, the gels were non-negotiable. They were one of the few things I could eat pain free, as well as stomach consistently, and they kept my energy and electrolyte levels steady when everything else was unpredictable. As time went on, I was struggling to eat real food and was relying more heavily on gels than I had anticipated. The crew leapt into action. A post went out on Facebook – an SOS to anyone following the run: 'Does anyone have Precision Hydration gels? We're running low.' Meanwhile, the team started raiding every health food shop they could find in nearby towns. Most hadn't even heard of the brand, and those that had just shook their heads apologetically.

Then came the miracle. A local legend called Sam replied to the post, saying he had a stash at home and could meet us. He drove out to what can only be described as the middle of nowhere, pulling up beside the van with a bag of gels like it was the most normal thing in the world (Precision Hydration kindly topped him up afterwards). I'll never forget that moment. It wasn't just about the gels. It was about people showing up. A stranger, watching from afar, choosing to step in and keep me going. When everything felt raw and vulnerable, that simple act of kindness reminded me why I was doing this—not just to break a record, but to connect people, to bring communities together in ways I could never have imagined.

By the early evening on day two I had hit the halfway mark, having covered 280km. My A goal was sub-80 hours, with my secondary target to finish under Mimi's time of 87.5 hours. My pacing gave me enough time to allow for something to go wrong and still break the record. Up until now I had been precisely on target, the 80-hour goal within reach.

But as I reached 290km my goal started to slip away. By 11 p.m. I was 18 minutes behind schedule. The unforgiving camber of Irish country roads had finally taken its toll, exacerbating an old knee injury. I had been running for 39 hours, most of it on the left-hand side of the road so Kate could cycle behind me. Subsequently my left leg was constantly slightly lower than my right, taking more of the strain, which was exactly what I'd dealt with in Spartathlon. Panic surged momentarily – I worried this was the end. My knee was so swollen it had doubled in size, but Kate sprang into action again, finding a knee support while the crew crudely strapped my knee in pink kinesiology tape. I necked a couple of paracetamols and continued, each step a little more cautious and calculated than before.

Night two was terrifying. By 1 a.m. deep exhaustion had set in, amplified by the relentless cold, rain and inky darkness. Having not slept on night one, my mind was clouded, slipping into a frightening, disorientated haze. The steady roar of heavy trucks rumbling past at terrifying speeds made my heart race and sent panic reverberating through my tired body. The road had narrowed, leaving no space to safely navigate, and with no hard shoulder available I felt dangerously exposed. Kate cycled beside me, valiantly attempting to shield us both, her figure illuminated like a Christmas tree by reflective gear and flashing lights. Yet even her reassuring presence felt small against the intimidating force of huge vehicles thundering by at 100km/h, their head-lights slicing aggressively through the dark. Each passing truck intensified my anxiety, my feet growing unsteady beneath me. I had lost track of exactly where we were, and the surroundings blurred into a nightmarish confusion.

The persistent drizzle combined with plunging temperatures chilled me to the bone. I desperately wanted to lie down, but instinctively knew collapsing on to the sodden grass would mean risking hypothermia. I had to keep going. By now the hallucinations were in full force. Shapes emerged from the shadows, vivid and disturbingly real. I saw witches' hats and glistening seaweed scattered across the road, the pointed silhouettes stark and eerie. As I swerved to avoid them, Kate glanced over, clearly concerned. I described what I was seeing, hoping desperately she'd confirm they were real. Instead, she admitted seeing something entirely different – and less haunting. 'Can you see all the rabbits bounc-ing around? And the stars falling down from the sky?' asked Kate. We exchanged a knowing look, the truth dawning grimly: if we were seeing entirely different visions, none of them could be real. This offered some comfort as the surreal scenes intensified, culminating in a fully lit nativity scene glowing red and green in the darkness of a town called Borrisokane.

We called the crew, waking them from a deep sleep. We both needed somewhere to stop and rest. I stumbled on, an audible moan coming from deep within my body. A moan of agony, and pain and fatigue. I just wanted to lie down. But the crew were struggling to find somewhere to park. Every step was becoming an excruciating ordeal. By now I'd run more than 320km and my body was at its limit. Mercifully, we finally saw the crew's camper van parked up ahead. Relief flooded through me as I stumbled towards its dimly lit interior and fell into the back, Kate cuddled beside me. Someone quickly draped a Dryrobe over me while someone else handed me a caffeine gel. I sucked it down automatically. For 20 precious minutes I slept dreamlessly beneath that dry robe. When Nick gently nudged me awake the caffeine was already beginning to surge through my veins, chasing away the fog. I sat up stiffly, reaching for a Red Bull to amplify the buzz. I shuffled along the road, the dry robe still wrapped over me, before dropping it on the roadside for the crew to collect. I knew the worst had passed, but the night had left a permanent mark making me realise just how fragile, vulnerable and exposed I really was.

Day three arrived with a buzz of anticipation that felt entirely different from the grinding uncertainty of the previous night. As dawn broke I could already feel the tempo quickening around me – the roads were busier, the support more vibrant and there was a growing sense of excitement as we edged closer to County Cork, the place I'd come to think of as a second home. The weather was kinder too, the rain subsiding and leaving behind a gusty wind. It was a day filled with relentless activity, a carousel of faces appearing and disappearing beside me as I continued south. I had only announced the challenge on social media 10 days before setting off, wanting to keep the pressure off until the very last minute, but word had spread quickly and tens of thousands of people were tracking my progress. By mid-morning I had covered 378km and there was a constant stream of beeping cars, homemade signs and waves from locals.

With just 57 minutes' sleep in the past 48 hours, I clung on to any stimulation I could. My sister-in-law Karen and a group of her friends joined me, injecting fresh energy into my run exactly when I needed it most. Karen, thoughtful as ever, had brought along a bar of Dairy Milk – simple, comforting and perfectly timed. I was struggling to eat and a sweet, smooth, chocolate treat was exactly what I craved in that moment. Running alongside Karen and her friends, listening to their lively chatter, was incredibly comforting. I'd reached the point where words felt exhausting, so instead I listened, quietly absorbing their conversations about everyday life, their children, funny stories from their week. Despite the enormity of the challenge, these miles felt surprisingly normal – just like an ordinary girls' run on any given day. It was reassuring to experience this gentle slice of normality amidst the extraordinary.

The highlight of my day came in the early afternoon, as I approached the school in County Limerick that symbolised the powerful impact of my run. From a distance, I could hear the growing noise of excited voices, chants and cheers carrying towards me. As I turned the corner, the sight before me was overwhelming: scores of schoolchildren lining the road, waving handmade banners and calling my name with genuine joy. My heart swelled and tears blurred my vision. The kids ran alongside me, their enthusiasm infectious, their laughter and shouts propelling me forward. It was an extraordinary moment, impossible to adequately capture in words, leaving me deeply emotional. I felt embraced by Ireland, fully adopted by this community in a way I'd never imagined.

Soon after, we reached the town of Killmallock, a place with deep personal connections to John's family. I ran past the house John's father was born in, and later, while sharing stories post run with John, I learned of a distant relative – another John

Power – who lived in a farm nearby. It was just the type of random family connection I was longing for on this journey.

Approaching the town, I spotted a familiar group gathered by the roadside – John's extended family, beaming with pride, and there, unexpectedly amid them all, was Saoirse. Seeing her small, eager face waiting to greet me filled my heart, even if I didn't have the energy to express it. High-fiving her tiny hand as I ran past was a powerful reminder of exactly why I'd undertaken this immense journey. It wasn't just a run – it was about family, connection and inspiring my daughter to see what she could one day achieve herself. I never envisaged that my challenge would also bring John's family together, but there were his parents, aunts and uncles, cheering me on and ringing ahead to the local schools to tell them I was coming.

It wasn't just John's family who were connected by the experience. Over in the UK something peculiar was happening. I'd always known that my parents weren't particularly interested in my running. It was not something they'd ever engaged with or supported, and over the years I'd never expected anything else. When I received eight A★s and an A in my GCSEs, my dad asked me why I got an A. It was upgraded later, but he noted it couldn't have therefore been a high A★. From that young age I felt freed from all parental expectation, knowing nothing I ever did – no exam or career success, athletic performance or advocacy would ever be 'enough', so I could set my own path in life. There was, however, a quiet sadness that sometimes caught me at races, especially when I saw other runners' parents – people in their 70s – standing patiently at checkpoints, sometimes in the middle of the night, clutching flasks of tea, and ready to hand out snacks and encouragement. My dad came to an ultra once to pick me up, but waited in the car as I crossed the line.

My parents both worked long hours to provide for my brother and I, so I was a latchkey kid, independent from a young age, and that sense of having to rely on myself became the foundation for my resilience. Everything I'd done, from applying to universities, to driving my career, to choosing this path of ultrarunning and advocacy, I'd done without a guiding hand. In many ways that parental absence had shaped me. It had made me tougher, more self-reliant, probably much more successful, but not immune to longing for a little more from my parents; so when I found out later that during the run across Ireland they had been tracking me online, it meant something. I hadn't realised at the time, but at one point my dad messaged John to say the battery on my tracker was running low and asked him to make sure I switched it over. It was such a small thing, but it showed me they were there in the background, watching quietly – not cheering from the sidelines with placards and warm drinks, but still present in their own way. Knowing they were following me, watching over me, was enough to warm a part of me that had been conditioned to expect nothing.

Passing through Charleville at 2 p.m. on day three I noticed the schedule was starting to slip. It was impossible to run on the downhills as my knee was sending sharp stabbing pains throughout my body. It was frustrating. I was an hour behind my 80-hour goal and yet it still seemed tantalisingly close. My spirits soared briefly as I glanced at one of my watches and the distance ticked below 100 miles (I was monitoring the run in miles).

Wearing two watches was essential. One stored my music and showed my pace while the other acted as navigation. There was so much data to capture that having two recording devices ensured we were covered. Everything down to my precise cadence would be analysed by Guinness, to verify another person hadn't run with my watch or to confirm I hadn't been given a lift in the van. On my right wrist was an Enduro displaying a large map and the distance to go. It ticked down from 558km like a never-ending countdown. I couldn't work out how to change the screen and didn't want to risk the data capture, so I was constantly faced with a huge screaming figure. When it eventually ticked over into double digits I squealed in delight.

As the miles rolled by, the reality of having to face a third night sank in. I had been snatching the odd 10-minute nap on the roadside, but I knew the sleep demons would be out in droves come sundown. John, always intuitive, recognised my growing need for his support as we approached what was likely to be another long, difficult night. He quietly decided to take the boys back to his parents' home and returned to join the crew.

As I trudged along, nervously anticipating the sunset, I reflected on day three. I felt a wave of gratitude. It had been a relentless day – hectic, loud, emotional – but deeply rewarding. Each beep, cheer, conversation and piece of chocolate had propelled me forward. The spontaneous support from communities along the way was a testament to the warmth of the Irish people. With nightfall approaching, my whole body in pain, but my heart full, I braced myself, confident and hopeful, ready to face whatever lay ahead.

Night three was a blur. I don't remember much about it – and maybe that's a mercy. I had a string of short naps, each one lasting 10 or 20 minutes. When the fatigue hit me hardest, I'd ask Kate to call ahead to the crew with the code: 'Get the hotel ready.' That was our euphemism for laying out the blow-up mattress on the side of the road. The second I saw it, I'd belly-flop down and knock back a caffeine gel. We called it a caffeine nap as the hit would kick in after I woke. By then, I'd stopped registering the kilometres in any meaningful way. My body was running on instinct, every joint aching, every part of my skin rubbed raw by wind, rain and friction. The worst was the chafing on my backside, which was sore and seeping, something I hadn't entirely anticipated. I couldn't even feel my swollen knee anymore. The pain had been drowned out by the sheer volume of discomfort everywhere else.

Finally dawn broke. There was a stillness that morning that felt different. The sun cast a golden glow over the landscape. I hadn't seen a proper sunrise the whole trip – it had been too cloudy and wet. But now the light stretched across the hills, warming the road ahead. It was the last day. The end was close. Liza joined me for a stretch, her calm energy grounding me in the moment. I knew the record was in the bag. The crew were still a little unsure, nervously checking timings and whispering about pace, but I'd done the mental maths. Numbers were my safe place. When everything else felt chaotic, I found order in arithmetic. It calmed me. I knew exactly how much time I had, how much further I had to go, and I was completely confident – I'd break the record.

Music played constantly through my headphones; a play-list of Irish songs John's dad had loaded on to my Shokz headphones. They entertained me for a while, but I was still bleeding time, unable to run on the downhills. The 80-hour pacing plan had all but disappeared – I was now three hours behind schedule and getting slower. But I knew I could hike it to the end in record-breaking time.

Kate, who had been my shadow on the bike for days, finally passed out in the van. She was broken. While she had originally planned to just ride with me during the tricky night sections, the busy roads meant she'd been on her bike supporting me 20 hours a day. Her job had been so much harder than mine in many ways – staying alert through every mile, scanning the road constantly for hazards, protecting me from traffic, navi-gating our route, carrying my supplies. She gave everything to keep me safe and now her body was giving out. In her words, I was the horse that just whined when I was tired and needed to be fed, but she was the camel continually plodding onward until she dropped dead.

John took over while Kate rested, and we passed through Bantry – the final town en route. John started telling me I was behind time and needed to go quicker, but it was really because the school children at the next village were waiting to see me before home time. When I realised he was telling porky pies, my anger woke me up before the children's cheers gave me another huge boost.

There was just one road to follow now, which led all the way to my final destination – Mizen Head. Support came in waves. Local runner Marcus arrived to support. He was instantly dubbed 'Marcus the Mule' and took over carrying Kate's heavy rucksack, walking beside me, steady and dependable. Nick joined too, breaking into bursts of Irish songs, making me laugh with his ridiculous cheer just when I needed it.

This being Ireland, the weather had one final test for me. After three days of wind and rain, the sun decided to make a guest appearance – in full dazzling costume. It was getting hot. Too hot. My body started to overheat, unable to regulate itself. The crew were genuinely worried. I could barely eat and was on the verge of heat exhaustion. Sugary snacks from the previous three days had burnt the inside of my mouth and even my adored jam tortillas were now refusing to go down. Gels, Mr Whippy ice cream and Coke were all I could stomach. Every few miles the crew stopped to pour water over my head, stuffing ice under my cap to get my body temperature down and refilling my ice bandana. Every cold splash made me yelp as it hit the raw surface of my bum – but at this point it was the lesser of two evils. At one point a road closure prevented the crew from getting to me and they began panicking that I would start overheating once more. Somehow, I managed to keep shuffling forward. A phantom of my former self, weakly waving to cheering schoolchildren and mustering up all my energy to simply form a smile. I had to keep moving – no more time for sleep now. Two hours and 17 minutes of shut eye would have to be enough. I powered on. The kilometres came and went. My watch counter went lower. I could do this.

As evening arrived the temperature began to drop and I was on the final breathtaking stretch to Mizen Head. Rolling rocky hills opened out to vast beaches, the sea sparkling in the sinking light. The road wound up ahead, slithering towards the coastline, and I felt myself slowing just a little – not from exhaustion, but to take it in; to remember. In the last few miles, I listened to a voice note from Eddie, my coach. As her voice filled my ears, speaking words of belief and pride, I completely crumbled. Tears streamed down my face. Eddie always knew what to say. This challenge had been worth every painful step.

With less than a mile to go I desperately wanted it to be over. But at the same time, I didn't. I wanted to soak up every last second, imprint it on my memory, bank it there forever. I didn't want to rush those final few steps. It had been the longest 558km of my life – three days, twelve hours and eight minutes. Over three hours ahead of Mimi's record.

I turned the corner and there they were – my family. The kids. John. Everyone who mattered. I kissed the Mizen Head sign. Hugged my children tightly. No fanfare, no fireworks. Just the people I loved, a battered body and a mind full of memories. I knew thousands of people were following me online. The impact had been far greater than I could have ever hoped. Those schoolchildren in Limerick would be forever seared in my heart, but for now, all I craved were the simple things in life. Rest. Comfort. Silence. A proper toilet. I wandered over to the gift shop and was gifted a Mizen Head hoodie by the owner – soft, warm, low key. Exactly how I wanted it. But as usual my next thoughts turned to where the crew would be sleeping, and how the kids were doing. It was straight back into maternal mode. I'd had my adventure and it was time to get back to normal.

Coda: Challenge yourself

I never expected to find myself running 558km across Ireland in an attempt to break a world record, but this challenge became so much more than physical endurance. It was about discovering what I was truly capable of – and showing other women and girls that they could push themselves too. Battling pain, exhaustion and a sea of logistical hurdles, I learned the power of resilience and the importance of surrounding yourself with people who believe in you. This run was personal – connecting with my children's heritage, running 'home' to my daughter and proving that women can do hard things. I finished not just as a record breaker, but as someone newly convinced of her strength. And from that strength I found the confidence to encourage others; to say to them, 'Go on, challenge yourself. Step outside your comfort zone and you'll be amazed at what you find.'

12

THINK OUTSIDE THE BOX

48 Hour Treadmill Record

'You are crazy. How on earth are you doing this?' It was day two of my 48-hour treadmill world record attempt and Sir Mo Farah was questioning my sanity. I was too. My tongue was swollen, my attempts to nap had repeatedly failed and the researchers probing me were beginning to approach me with caution. Inside I was miserable. I was really struggling. But to the outside world I kept on smiling. I was on display after all. Leaning into the misery, I held firm. If Mo Farah, a multiple Olympic, World and European Champion was impressed by my running, then maybe this was something especially difficult.

The decision to attempt a treadmill record had ignited as I ran across Ireland. During that challenging journey I'd been deeply moved by the runners who came out to join me. Here I was running through the backroads of Ireland surrounded by others who wished to take on adventures of their own. I struck up amazing conversations with women who had never run more than a few miles before, and was surrounded by a whizz of school children as I ran through villages. They understood what I was doing and talked eagerly about challenging themselves.

The message of self-empowerment was getting through, but I had only just scratched the surface. What if there was a way for more people to see this? In the quieter periods when I ran for hours in rural solitude, I took time to reflect. I found myself craving something different – something public, something people could truly engage with on a larger scale. I wanted to reach a wider community. A plan started to formulate.

As I tossed and turned restlessly in bed during the sleepless nights that always followed a physical event like this, everything started to come together. I had a lot of boxes I wanted to tick; I wanted a challenge that tested me in a different way. I'm not one to do the same race or event time and again, chasing new PBs. I leapt straight into ultrarunning so I never had those standard 5k, 10k, marathon targets in my mind. I couldn't even tell you what my fastest 5k time was. I had wanted to run Spartathlon again, but since Ireland my goals had shifted and my Sparta journey seemed less important. All that was important to me right now was impact – to reach as many people as possible to inspire, empower and demonstrate what women are all truly capable of.

Attempting another world record seemed like the obvious choice. Regularly competing internationally was difficult due to family logistics. An overseas race would mean being away from my children and complex arrangements for my support crew. I had already leaned heavily on friends and family for my Ireland record. I didn't want to keep asking favours or to be a burden to others, and I had no sponsorship to cover costs. If I tackled another world record it needed to be on home turf and super-practical to do. Setting records also involves a lot of bureaucracy. This is absolutely necessary to ensure records are verified and validated, but it takes a lot of work. Witnesses must be found, which can be extremely tricky when you are running on a remote country road at 3 a.m. I had to think outside the box to achieve all my criteria and minimise my daily juggle.

Despite my immense fatigue, recovery brought a sense of clarity as the idea solidified. One of the benefits of being an unsponsored athlete was that I could focus on challenges that really made my heart sing. I had no obligation to run in specific races or to compete in the same events as my peers. I could do exactly what I wanted and at this particular point in my running career I wanted meaningful impact. If I could set up a treadmill somewhere public, I would have audience reach and it would be far easier for a crew to support. There would be thousands of witnesses on hand. Everything would be in one place.

I started googling treadmill world records. As ridiculous as it sounds, 24 hours seemed like too comfortable a distance. I performed better over longer distances, as we'd found out in the World Championships when I'd started overtaking runners towards the end. I wanted to see what I could achieve over a longer stretch of time. The current female world record for 48 hours on a treadmill was 340km. I knew I could run 236km in 24 hours on a track, and very naively thought a treadmill would be easier, so I thought I would just go a bit slower than that and then walk the rest. It seemed possible, so without further consideration I settled on the idea of a 48-hour record – I just needed a venue.

In seven months' time it would be the National Running Show, housed inside a series of colossal warehouse-type buildings at the Birmingham National Exhibition Centre (NEC). It was only a 90-minute drive from my home in Surrey. It gave me enough time to recover from Ireland and get back to peak condition. It was far enough away from the 24 Hour World Championships in October 2025 and the date fitted into my training calendar perfectly. Just 10 days after finishing the Ireland record, I fired off an email to Mike Seaman, a good friend of mine and also the director of the National Running Show: 'Had a crazy idea in one of my multiple daily naps… I'm looking at breaking the world record for 48 hrs on a treadmill and January seems like the best timing (this hasn't even gone to my coach yet though). Ideally it's in a controlled temperature lab… But might the run show work?'

After a nervous week of silence, I received Mike's reply: 'Love this idea and have actually been trying to make something like this work at the Running Show for ages – just needed someone to do it!!!' There was no turning back. I had seven months to prepare.

Handling logistics was my phenomenal friend Kate Strong, who had supported me on her bicycle across the whole of Ireland. She had previously broken the world record for the greatest distance covered on a static bike in 24 hours and knew how to deal with the paperwork. Working with Kate Jamieson, head of content at the National Running Show, she did everything, from finding a crew of volunteers, to securing 17 witnesses to sign paperwork every two hours, to sourcing tens of thousands of calories, worth of diverse nutrition, music, cooling fans and an inflatable bed. For insurance purposes I also needed my own St John Ambulance crew member on hand for the full 48 hours, plus a security guard, and this was all handled impeccably by the National Running Show team. Without them and Kate Strong, none of it would have been possible. I didn't have to arrange a thing. My only job was to turn up and run. The National Running Show was logistically feasible and reasonably easy to support, but was an environment that would be chaotic and hot, where I would be under constant public scrutiny. Still, it felt right. I had the dual goal of pushing myself to an untested limit and maximising public engagement. Ironically, thinking outside the box would lead me to running inside a giant metal one.

With the event confirmed, reality quickly sank in. I was not in peak shape. The aftermath of Ireland had left my knee severely injured. Recovery had been slow, compounded by unexpectedly low iron levels. I'd discovered the iron deficiency via a blood test after weeks of struggling with inexplicable fatigue. No matter how many chocolate brownies I ate I felt chronically exhausted.

I should have rested, but instead a pre-booked family holiday saw me competing in the challenging Sur les Traces des Ducs de Savoie (TDS) race in Chamonix that August, while the kids and John enjoyed relaxing hikes in the mountains. Though beautiful, it was a punishingly technical 148km race in harsh conditions. Part of the incentive to do this event was that Alexis Berg, who had taken the viral photograph of me breastfeeding Cormac at UTMB, had promised to take a photo of me and the kids at the end of the race. Saoirse, my youngest who was just three at the time, kept asking why she wasn't in any of my race finisher pictures. This ate away at me and my visualisation for the race became the family photo at the end.

With my knee heavily strapped I took on the course, which had an elevation gain of 9300m, knowing I shouldn't really be there. From the very beginning I felt uncomfortable. It was 11 p.m., pitch black, and I was tightly penned into the starting area, pushed up against a sea of male bodies, not able to even see another woman. When I bent down to tie my shoelace someone took the opportunity to grope my arse. The pen was so densely populated and it was so dark I couldn't tell who it was. This was not the freedom of trail running that I loved. It felt more like cattle being herded to the slaughter. I felt frightened and helpless to do anything. There was no protocol, no-one to report it to and sadly it was an all-too-common occurrence. There was medical protection on the race but no way to prevent women from being harassed. The safeguarding fell woefully short, which I made a mental note of to address with SheRACES for all events.

Finally, the starting horn sounded and we shuffled off into the dark. Soon the feeling of discomfort turned to frustration. I was faster on the steep uphill climbs, but many runners blocked me from passing, putting their poles out wide as a barrier. On the descents I tried to keep to the side, but was still pushed out of the way on multiple occasions, the men down in 300+ position clearly needing to make up places. The declines put a huge amount of stress on my knee, with my weight pushing down on it, while marching up the inclines relieved the stress. It was a race of polar opposites and I dreaded the downhills. As a result, despite the majestic remote mountains, I enjoyed very little of the race, with much of it spent clambering over endless boulders cursing my lack of technical experience.

An additional stress was my heavy period, for which there was inadequate race support. It wasn't an A race, so I didn't reschedule my period, letting my cycle run naturally, but there were no period products available on the course, and I quickly ran out of mine. The year before I had discussed the need for period product provision with UTMB, the race organisers of TDS, in my director role at SheRACES. They had promised these would be provided, yet at every aid station they were missing or inadequate. To add insult to injury, men were using the women's toilets, despite there being hardly any queue at the men's, and staff refused my request to police them. The only place to change out of my wet clothes was the sink area of the toilet, which added to my frustration, and that of the women around me. I needed space to take off my bra and attend to my chafing using the mirror to guide me, but men kept piling into the toilet.

Still in recovery from my Irish crossing I was tired of running and tired of fighting for change. But I made it through to Chamonix where I forgot all about the pain and frustration as I ran through the streets with all three children, them taking in the atmosphere and enjoying the cheers. Alexis was waiting on the finish line as promised, capturing the moment for Saoirse. It had been a tough race and the technical terrain did not play to my strengths, but at least I could now relax with my family and friends. After the TDS, rather than put my feet up, I had a long meeting with the operations director of UTMB to ensure women in the rest of the races that week didn't have to go through the same difficulties that I had.

Putting the TDS behind me I threw myself back into training. The National Running Show were keen to announce the world record attempt, but I kept pressing pause. I wasn't ready to go public yet. I decided to enter one of my favourite November races to test my fitness. The Wendover Woods is a 80km looped ultra through the Chilterns in the south of England run by Centurion. It consists of five 16km loops through enchanting forest trails during the cusp of autumn. Runnable climbs and smooth descents are mixed with juicy steep sections scattered along the course. It is usually ideal running conditions, being soft underfoot, during a cool but not frigid part of the year, and with two checkpoints per loop I knew I could escape if something went wrong.

The first few hours went perfectly. I was having the time of my life, flying down the beautiful soft trails covered with a loose dusting of leaves. I was cautiously optimistic, lapping up every loop. Then just under 50km in my knee suddenly went again. I tried to run on, but it didn't feel right. It was time to pull out. This was not my most important race of the year, where I would limp to the end before taking time off to recover. It was a day out to run at a good pace and get some miles in the legs. I was comfortable with a DNF, because it was necessary to prevent further damage. I had my eyes on the prize, and I wasn't going to blindly continue just for the sake of finishing this race. As in Courmayeur, I had got what I came for (in that case, marmots). I had banked some miles, escaped my head for the day, and there was no need to push through the pain. Wendover became a catalyst for renewed focus and my resolve solidified. It was time to get strong again.

The training build didn't exactly go according to plan, though, with the injury flare-up at Wendover halting some of my runs. By October 2024 I had been base training around 80 to 95km per week, but this dropped dramatically to 40km following the race DNF. However, as I passed through late November and into early December, and my knee started to feel better, I picked up the distance to around 100 or 105km per week, plus two strength workouts and two mobility sessions. I mostly avoided the treadmill, instead choosing to go for long flat runs close to home. I was deliberately avoiding the mental horror of the treadmill – burying my head over how hard it would be. My only endurance session on the treadmill was a one-off four-hour run (Eddie proposed a six-hour one which was met with a strong pushback!). I didn't really want to know what the monotony would feel like – I would just face it when I had to.

With my strength training, I focused on upper body strength with Brendan (my strength coach), particularly my neck. I knew this had a tendency to collapse over time and lifting weights with my neck had prepared me well for Ireland (with the help of my osteo Gunter Knockaert at Club La Santa). We also worked on my core, which I'd need to keep me steady, working up to

25kg dumbbells for my renegade rows, where you plank holding on to dumbbells and pull each upwards in turn.

By the Christmas holidays I was back on track. Literally. Our annual family tradition is to spend the fortnight break at Club La Santa, an active holiday resort in Lanzarote. We visit both sets of grandparents the week before, and then head off for some winter sun. While Santa does come (on Christmas Eve, as it's Spain), he can only leave a small (sports-related, of course) present so we avoid child-led demands for 'stuff'. The children get to scale large ladders to dress the huge hotel Christmas tree while parents drink mulled wine. On Christmas day they open their stockings, which every year include dive toys, goggles/sunglasses/sports bottles to replace ones they've already lost, and enough Haribo to fuel their sporting escapades for the next week. By 10 a.m. on Christmas morning it's all over and we're off for a family game of padel/pickleball/badminton.

While the kids were in a variety of sports classes and activities in Club La Santa, I racked up distances on the hotel running track and local trails, reaching 145+km per week, alongside a multitude of functional classes and HYROX races (HYROX combines functional strength exercises with running). This was my final reprieve, my go-no-go testing ground. I either pulled the plug on my world record attempt or ploughed full steam ahead. Sneaking out early one morning while the kids were still asleep, I hit the track for a 50k run-easy session. This was my four-hour fitness litmus test. It had served me well before the 24 Hour World Championships as a test of my fitness levels.

I love track running at La Santa. It is the perfect place to watch the world go by, from taking in the sunrise, to seeing the same people on their way to the daily morning gymnastics, then the daily 5km group run, then out to various fitness classes, before wandering back and wondering why that crazy woman is still running around the track. During this particular session, when the boys finally woke up they joined a football class on the pitch, so I could see them as I looped around, before watching them play padel on the courts. My friend Dame Sarah Storey was recovering from an ankle injury so came to cheer, crew (and laugh at me) as she did her daily rehab sessions in the sunshine. I ran in the outside lane, changing direction every hour, wearing an old GB vest which always seems to make people clear a lane for me. Sprinters lined up on the straights doing their drills, then zoomed past me, making me feel very slow indeed.

I clipped along at a pace of 4:52 minutes per kilometre, knowing I had a deadline to meet, but needing it to feel as effortless as possible. I had a bet with Conrad, one of the sports instructors known as the Green Team, that after my 50km I'd make it to his functional fitness class at 11 a.m. – and of course I did. My stubbornness meant that having made the bet there was no way I was going back on it. Though it felt like madness at the time, the post-run session kept me moving, aiding my recovery. Double workout complete, I felt strong and ready. My body was finally in shape. It was the affirmation I needed. I'd passed the test. With three weeks to go it was time to press the button and announce the treadmill challenge. I was ready.

Wanting to squeeze every opportunity out of my record bid, I decided it was a prime time to become a medical guinea pig. This was a chance not just to test my limits, but to advance scientific research into women's endurance. I contacted Dr Jamie Pugh from Liverpool John Moores University, who had previously supported me at the European Championships and was a key advisor for the GB 24-hour team. Jamie was both a scientist and an experienced ultrarunning crew member, making him ideal to lead the research. He was extremely supportive and quickly assembled a team of student scientists. This collaboration was vital. Research on female endurance athletes remains minimal – only 6 per cent of sports science studies focus exclusively on women. And for the studies that do include both men and women, only a third of the data is collected from female participants. The team conducted extensive testing, including cognitive assessments, blood lactate measurements, gut health monitoring and hourly gas oxidation analyses to capture comprehensive physiological data throughout my treadmill attempt. They also took bloods before and after the event to send to the company Thriva to analyse any changes. Knowing the science team were relying on my data gave me the extra motivation to keep moving when things got tough. I now had three powerful elements to my 'why': to test my limits, to inspire others and to inform scientific study. It was time to tread.

Baked beans. Why on earth did I choose baked beans as my final meal before running non-stop for two days? Several hours into my treadmill challenge and I was regretting my life choices. It had all started promisingly the night before with a calorific meal of pizza and cake. I was staying at a hotel close to the NEC in the Midlands, where the National Running Show is held each January. I managed a luxurious lie-in on the morning of the record attempt before eating a traditional English breakfast of sausages, toast, hash browns and troublesome baked beans. Topping up my carbs at lunchtime I had my tried-and-tested bowl of porridge and banana, but it was too late – the beans were brewing.

Arriving at 1.30 p.m. I entered the vast maze of corrugated rectangular buildings dressed in a fetching hi-viz jacket. Inside the air was cool and still, but there was already a thrum of activity as exhibitors prepared for the show. I was beginning my challenge at 2.30 p.m. on Friday 24 January 2025, 19 hours before the public arrived and the show officially opened on the Saturday. Assessing my baseline cognitive function pre-attempt, the science team placed an iPad in my hands and conducted a series of tests. The games involved memorising words and numbers, and mind tricks like clicking the colour of the text rather than the word it spelt. My bloods had already been taken in the morning and I knew the team would be taking constant readings throughout.

As I stepped on to the treadmill, the lights of the NEC buzzed brightly around me. I could see banners being raised, stalls being assembled, and the steady trickle of show personnel moving in and out of the vast hall. A large sign for the running shoe company Salomon loomed in my direct line of sight. Knowing I'd stare at this for days felt both intimidating and strangely comforting – this was my world now; my challenge, my choice.

Stepping onto the treadmill I took a deep breath, checked my team were ready, and pressed the start button. I heard a few gentle claps echo in the empty hall and put my head down. I desperately tried not to think about what was ahead of me. It was just another treadmill run. I swiftly got into the zone, mesmerised by the spectacle growing before my eyes. The kilometres ticked by comfortably and my spirits remained high. Inquisitive individuals came by to ask what I was doing and my crew, led by Kate Strong and Jamie's researchers, rotated frequently. I watched as they busily problem solved, finding fans to keep me cool, locating a WiFi code to enable me to watch TV, and working out the best position for my nutrition. To keep my mind occupied I listened to the *Tea and Trails* podcast co-hosted by my coach Eddie Sutton. She was meant to come down to run with me during the first night on the companion treadmill to my left, but a storm had left her stranded in Scotland. I was gutted, but listening to her voice provided some comfort.

My strategy was to run the first day at just under my usual 24-hour race strategy. This meant eight three-hour slots, starting at a pace of 11.3km/h, but getting slightly slower with each block. I was moving consistently and everything was going well until the early evening, when my tummy began hurting and the beans went into full evacuation mode.

Between sprints to the toilet the pain continued to crescendo, akin to labour contractions every few minutes. Fortunately, the treadmill had been set up right next to the loos, meaning I wasted little time travelling back and forth as my guts continually cramped. Like a scene out of a TV hospital drama, every time I wanted to use the toilet, a crew member rushed to the disabled loo, which was the closest, clutching an emergency box, and shouted, 'Clear!' After waiting for the treadmill to completely stop, which seemed to take an age, I then jogged to the cubicle and rummaged through the box, which contained wet wipes, hand sanitiser, lip balm, hair grips and chafing cream.

However, unbeknownst to me there was chaos going on behind the scenes. The treadmill had only arrived in position 20 minutes before I started. Kate had planned to have at least two hours to test the machine, learn its quirks and get prepared. None of this happened. As evening arrived and I was dashing back and forth to the toilet it became apparent that the treadmill was resetting itself. If there was too long a pause the mileage reset to zero. Kate had no idea this would happen. This could jeopardise the entire record. As panic rose from the pit of Kate's stomach, she told me everything was under control: they were not only keeping a log of all the mileage, but it was saved on the treadmill operating system. Her job was to keep me calm, focused and completely oblivious. I had no idea anything was wrong, but it was very wrong indeed.

The video footage was capturing me running, but it wasn't capturing the treadmill screen, which showed the accumulated mileage and thus the distance I'd run. This would not be enough evidence for Guinness, but fortunately, every time I came off the treadmill, witnesses had been meticulously photographing the screen and doing the same again when I stepped back on. These photos clinched the world record confirmation, and without them Guinness would have rejected the attempt. However, because there was no ongoing mileage on the treadmill screen, Kate was constantly hunting down witnesses to check their photos so she could add up the mileage total. I was completely unaware any of this was happening. I just kept plodding forward as the stall holders gradually headed off for a relaxing evening before the show opened the next day. The main lights were gradually switched off and I was left under the glow of a strip of fluorescent ceiling lights.

At 11 p.m, two Running Show ambassadors (there to help promote the show on social media) wandered in, curious to see how I was doing. They had been to the pub for dinner and thought they'd pop by to say hello. They ended up staying for three hours, running 20km on the second treadmill set up next to me, in jeans and 'fashion' trainers. They were overheating like mad, but the hilarity of the surreal situation kept me going. By 12.10 a.m. I had passed 100km. I was now almost 10 hours into the challenge and my stomach was starting to settle down. One technical aspect that made a huge difference was using a glucose monitor. The team had hooked me up to a Libre Glucose sensor on my arm before the start. When I began feeling nauseous after quickly taking down a 90-gram gel – which I'd nicknamed the 'antisocial' because it usually meant the crew could leave me alone for over an hour – I checked my glucose levels on my phone, which connected to the sensor via Bluetooth. By tracking my blood sugar in real time, I was able to delay eating again until my levels dropped, giving my stomach nearly two hours to settle. That simple piece of tech helped me manage my nutrition better, made me feel significantly less sick, and allowed me to continue fuelling effectively throughout the challenge.

The plan was always to set off at a strong pace, so I had more time to play with on the second day when I was reaching the unknown of what my body could handle. But every three hours the crew would nudge my pace down slightly, so it became more manageable once the expo officially opened and the public – and their distractions – arrived. Sleep was out of the question as my body didn't know how to switch off under the unnaturally bright fluorescent lights, but I did manage a five-minute lie down. Wrestling with the blow-up bed next to the treadmill, I pulled on my eye mask and slid under a blanket. It was just about enough rest to refresh my body before starting over, but my mind was still struggling with the constant surveillance. I felt uneasy knowing every single move was being recorded on video and in person. Two of my eight-person crew were constantly by my side – even during these brief rests – acting as timekeepers for Guinness, working on four-hour shifts. Then every two hours two independent witnesses had to come and sign a statement – a total of 20 people over the entire record attempt. Some of these were friends, but many of them were strangers to me – random people Kate had persuaded to help. Being watched made it hard to truly relax; I was craving privacy even in the middle of the night, yet fully aware that solitude wasn't part of what I had signed up for. I was beginning to realise this would be a far greater mental challenge than a physical one – and I had completely underestimated how draining it would be to remain so visible throughout.

The contrast the next morning was staggering. With no daylight filtering in, my only sense of time came from movements within the hall. It started to fill up as first the exhibitors and then the public began filing into the space. The hum of activity was energising, uplifting me as friends and professional athletes came by to say hello. A pep talk by American ultra-running legend Scott Jurek early on Saturday morning was just what I needed. He came behind the white picket fence separating me from the public and chatted about the ridiculousness of what I was doing, which was so much harder than being out solo on the trails. Being able to talk honestly to someone who knew what I was going through meant I was able to take off the veneer for a few minutes – a welcome mental relief. By the time British Olympians Colin Jackson and Sir Mo Farah strolled over to offer words of encouragement, I was flying. There was a constant stream of visitors and I had lovely, monotony-busting conversations with runners Jasmin Paris, Emma Stuart, Nicky Spinks, Anna Harding, Jo Pavey, Jenni Falconer, Spencer Matthews and 'Hardest Geezer' Russ Cook, who, even though he had run 9900 miles across Africa, was seemingly in awe of the mental challenge I was undertaking.

Some of the moments I cherished most were when members of the public signed up to run alongside me. Equally special was watching Kate tack homemade signs, crafted by children, on to the white picket fence in front of me. The collective energy of the crowd, friends and fellow athletes visiting initially kept me buoyed, but as the hours passed, temperatures inside the show rose significantly, exacerbated by thousands of attendees crowding the hall. Sweat was streaming down my face and the stuffy air, combined with the lack of any sort of breeze, became intolerable. My crew employed ice, wet towels and fans to cool me down, but overheating became a growing concern. I shoved a handful of ice cubes down my bra as my physical discomfort intensified. I had nowhere to hide.

The environment was relentless – bright lights, constant noise, crowds watching closely. I felt like an animal at the zoo. All my plans of watching television went out the window. I had stored up the whole of series three of *The Traitors* to binge – and warned everyone not to tell me what happened! But unlike my usual treadmill workouts I couldn't concentrate on the screen, because there was too much going on. Instead, the crew blasted music and questionable playlists through a pair of speakers in an attempt to keep me energised.

I always knew conditions at the National Running Show would not be ideal – and it was proving to be true. It was too hot and too busy and on Saturday, halfway into the record, I was struggling. Being on show with no escape from public gaze was stifling – compounded by the literally lifeless air. More failed attempts at 20-minute naps followed and I grew increasingly frustrated. Trying to lie down to rest just wasted time if I couldn't actually grab a few minutes' sleep. The pressure built up silently inside me. I was desperate not to take it out on my crew – I was so grateful for the time they had given up – but hiding my anguish made everything so much harder, because there was no way to release the pressure. Each time the science team stuck a mask on my face or drew some blood I inwardly (and probably outwardly) glared at them. These tests were becoming annoying and felt increasingly invasive, but I had to hold it together. My legs were fine, but I needed mental rest. The toilet became my refuge. It was the only place I could escape to for privacy and solace. It was impossible to nap next to the treadmill because of the lights and noise. When I desperately needed respite, I slipped off to rest on the toilet seat and simply close my eyes.

Sleep was not the only debilitating factor. Twenty-four hours into the challenge and my tongue was swollen. Despite those early stomach issues, I'd been on top of my nutrition, eating at regular intervals. Jam sandwiches, chews, jelly babies, jelly beans and Haribo were my reliable foods of choice. But by the middle of Saturday my mouth was burning from all the fruit and sugar. I had to switch to bananas and sports gels, as they were the only things I could swallow. These were washed down with Red Bull and Coca Cola, which I could still stomach. I managed to keep sipping water and electrolytes, and made random food requests as cravings popped into my head – at one point munching on a piece of mango.

As I sweated away, I longed for the evening when the show would be closed and I could savour the quiet once more; but peace would have to wait. As the last of the public trundled out into the early evening, they were replaced by a raucous National Running Show awards ceremony. It seemed to go on for an inordinate amount of time. I just wanted everyone to go home and leave me alone; yet when I heard huge cheers of 'Sophie, Sophie' coming from that direction, I felt such a boost knowing that hundreds of people were by my side.

At one point during the night, barefoot runner Vic Owens joined me and attempted to teach me a trick she called 'REM sleep' – closing your eyes and moving your eyeballs side to side for a few seconds to mimic REM sleep and supposedly trick the body into rest. I gave it a go during one of my many toilet breaks. I'm not sure it worked, but by that point I was willing to try anything. Also recognising that I might need a mental pick-up through the last night (and perhaps that my suffering was his fault, having said yes to the whole idea), Mike Seaman joined me post-awards ceremony at 2.30 a.m., running next to me and spilling out a stream of terrible (in the best possible way) jokes. It was going to be a long, hard, second night.

As the clocked ticked over into Sunday, I had been running non-stop for 34 hours. I'd only managed five minutes of actual sleep in that time (with many more failed nap attempts where I just couldn't nod off). The hallucinations began.

A mannequin on the nearby Harrier stand morphed into unsettling apparitions, a ghostly presence disrupting my fragile peace. It became my nemesis and I dreaded the very sight of it. This was not like outdoor racing. Whenever I have raced overnight outside, the sunrise has always been a rejuvenating moment. When that first chink of sunlight appears on the horizon you feel reborn. But stuffed inside a box under artificial lighting my body did not experience the same reprieve. The exhaustion and neurological sapping were unlike anything I have experienced before, but somehow I managed to get through the second night, and by 8 a.m. I had busted the previous record of 340km set by Emma Timmis. She is an incredible runner who also holds the seven-day treadmill record (no thanks!) and the fastest crossing of New Zealand on foot. She set a high bar and beating her record demanded every ounce of my strength.

It was time to have a nap. I managed 20 minutes of wonderful sleep before the show opened. I changed my clothes and tried to mentally prepare for the public gaze. As the doors opened at 9 a.m. I was still running, albeit at a slower pace than the day before. Suddenly a wave of disorientation washed over me and I panicked as I realised I could not run on the treadmill anymore. I could run to the toilet – solid ground was fine – but once I was back on that rotating floor my balance was thrown. I was bashing into the bars, and under Guinness World Record rules wasn't allowed to touch the treadmill to steady myself, but it was dangerous and I was convinced I was going to fall off. There was nothing I could do but switch to powerwalking. Thankfully the movement of hiking enabled me to recalibrate my balance. I was still ticking off the miles, but I wasn't running. It was at this point I regretted leaving John at home. He was looking after the kids and would bring them to the show for the final push later that day. As amazing as my crew were, I had a nagging feeling John would have been able to solve this problem with me, but John wasn't there, so I resigned myself to hiking it out as swiftly as I could – at 6km an hour.

With a repositioned focus, I seized the opportunity to soak up the atmosphere and chat to my well-wishers rather than tune out and hunker down. The record was in the bag and I could consciously absorb the impact I was making. I loved seeing the look on people's faces as they clocked the distance I had covered and asked questions about SheRACES. It also gave me the chance to properly chat with the runners beside me – something I hadn't always managed the day before, when I'd felt so rough I could barely get a word out. Another advantage of hiking was that I was finally able to have a cup of tea. I'd been longing for one, but hadn't managed to find a safe technique for drinking a cuppa while running, and I hadn't wanted to take a longer walking break before to do so. That first sip was divine.

With just four hours to go my family arrived, a fresh lease of life leaping on to the treadmill beside me. Three-year-old Saoirse had never been on a treadmill before, and I was spellbound as I watched her unnatural movements turn into a confident run. She grinned back at me as she realised she was running like mummy. It took my mind off the whole endeavour, away from the darkest moments, and towards the last stretch. I was nearly there.

A massive crowd had gathered round me as 2.30 p.m. approached on Sunday afternoon. Cheering crowds counted down as I closed in on the 48-hour marker. Out of the corner of my eye I spotted a BBC camera crew capturing my final steps. I was overwhelmed. The crowd began to cheer and clap excitedly. As the countdown began, I burst into tears. Just 10 more steps. Nine. Eight. Seven. Six. Five. Four. Three. Two. One. Stop. Stop. What just happened? I hugged Kate and then was almost knocked over by my kids, excited to have their mummy back. I had run 370.9km on a treadmill for two days. But it wasn't over yet. My blood was taken by the student crew, and minutes later I was whisked to the main stage to be interviewed by Susie Chan and Iwan Thomas in front of hundreds of Running Show attendees.

My three kids stood at the front jumping up and down, yelling 'Go Mummy,' while a stagehand ushered me into the spotlight, sliding a chair beneath me. Susie made a joke about the high stage stools being too perilous for me, before thrusting the mic towards me to ask how I felt. 'I'm quite tired. I can't wait for a nap,' I murmured through a hoarse throat. I was stuttering and slurring my words, but managed to stay just about with it, despite my mind frantically trying to process everything. 'It's such a crazy thing to do inside the NEC. Ultrarunning is usually a solo sport and to do the absolute opposite is so different. It has been such a unique experience.' I even managed to crack a couple of jokes and asked the audience not to tell me who had won *The Traitors*. With fatigue seeping in, colour draining from my cheeks, I held on to my why, pressing home the importance of breaking barriers in women's sport. Thanking all my supporters I stared at the crowd in a daze. Amazingly, I'd been able to make it to the stage without assistance. One benefit of switching to hiking during those penultimate hours was that it helped flush the lactic acid from my legs, preventing them from seizing up. Susie kindly wrapped the interview up quickly and I scuttled back to my crew.

The science team had one last final request. I had to repeat the cognitive test. This time I barely managed to answer any of the questions, at one point falling asleep while staring at the screen. My reaction time was so slow the computer programme thought I hadn't seen the questions. My brain was barely functioning. It was time to go home. Thinking ahead, Mike had secured John a pass allowing him to drive right up to the arena entrance (avoiding a 10-minute walk to the car park), where he bundled me and the kids straight into the car. I snoozed all the way home before falling straight into bed.

Monday morning arrived too soon and I was a mess. I had failed to eat upon leaving the NEC and now I couldn't face any food – not even a spoonful of my dad's phenomenal homemade chocolate ice cream. I knew not eating enough would delay my recovery, but it was days before my appetite returned. For now, I had to focus on getting the kids ready for school and answering requests for interviews. My friend Claire scooped up the boys, so I didn't have to face the steep hill to school. Once the kids were out of the door I collapsed in bed, John working from home to keep an eye on me. Pouring over my Garmin stats the enormity of what I had achieved began to sink in. With an average pace of 7:46 minutes per kilometre, including toilet stops and naps, and a typical heart rate of 116 beats per minute continually for 48 hours, my body had been pushed to the limit. Even my cadence had rarely slowed.

For the next few days I tried to take it easy, but work was piling up and there was admin to do. I wasn't a professional athlete. Elites are paid to nap, paid to have nine hours sleep a night and paid to do daily rehab. When they are resting their salary is still being paid, but I couldn't afford to take time off. I was back to mum duty, Zoom meetings and endless emails. I was juggling consultancy work, SheRACES development and booking in corporate speaking events. In an ideal world I would have taken the week off and retreated to a spa, but that wasn't possible. At least I had a break from running. I was under strict instructions from my coach Eddie to avoid all exercise other than walking. I closely monitored my heart rate variability, tried to eat and rest as much as a mum of three can, and vowed never to do a treadmill record attempt again.

As much as I admired people who returned to beat their previous records, I had not anticipated how mentally tough the challenge would be. Having no time to think, no personal space and people gawping at me all day was mentally draining. Smiling for selfies, waving at visitors and trying to look happy cost me an awful lot of energy. Post-record I was a washing machine of emotions, churned up inside. I would not have changed the crazy experience for the world and was so grateful to everyone who came to support me. I was happy to give the energy, but had not truly understood how hard it would be. It had put me off treadmill records for life.

As I reflected on the experience, my emotions were complex – a mix of pride, relief, frustration at not having pushed myself further, and overwhelming fatigue. I had achieved a world record and made a real impact, but I had wanted to keep running, to reach as close to 400km as possible. In the first 24 hours I was ahead of target and I was gutted when I had to revert to hiking. Unhelpful comments from a few passing Sunday spectators, overheard when I was 46 hours in to the attempt – like 'She's not even running' – kept whirring around in my head. My weakness is always hearing the one negative comment in a sea of a thousand supporters. I beat the record by 30km, but I knew inside I had the strength and fitness to do more. I just couldn't stay straight. And safe. I couldn't risk falling and not being able to walk the kids up the hill to school the week after.

But while I was frustrated at my body, what struck me most was discovering the depth of my mental resilience. Physically challenging as the treadmill record was, it was the psychological battle that had the greatest effect. I realised how deeply mental strength defines my identity as an athlete and person. I'm not genetically talented. I've just developed this mental and physical resilience over time. If I can do it then anyone can do it. This insight reshaped my self-perception, affirming that my most significant achievements might still lie ahead, even as I head towards perimenopause – because whenever the mind is more important than the body, I know I have an edge.

Coda: Think outside the box

Undertaking the 48-hour treadmill world record attempt forced me not just to push my physical limits, but to creatively overcome logistical hurdles and find innovative ways to inspire others. Initially, the decision to run on a treadmill at a public event felt counterintuitive – trapped in a literal and figurative box, exposed to constant scrutiny. Yet, ironically, stepping into that confined space expanded my impact far beyond anything I'd imagined. Throughout this journey, thinking outside the box meant recognising my priorities as a mother, athlete and advocate. It involved balancing ambition with the practicalities of family life, managing injury setbacks and leveraging the event to advance scientific understanding of female endurance. This approach brought immense personal clarity: embracing unconventional methods can unlock extraordinary outcomes.

13
PAY IT FORWARD

Road to the 24 Hour World Championships 2025

My inflammation markers were through the roof. It wasn't surprising since I'd been running on a treadmill for 48 hours, but they still made for sober reading. The blood testing company Thriva had been supporting the science study on my treadmill attempt and told me I had the 15th highest inflammation level out of over 48,000 blood tests in the company's database (that's the top 0.03 per cent). If their chief doctor didn't know how I had just spent my weekend, the results would be ringing alarm bells for a viral infection, auto-immune disease or even cancer. I would have been whisked off to accident and emergency, rather than encouraged to sit on the sofa and eat cake.

The test results post-world record attempt were telling me loud and clear that I needed to rest. It was a clear indication of the state of my nervous system and how much recovery I needed. Physically I was feeling pretty good and within a few days I felt ready to run again – which was why I needed the blood tests. Without them I would have been too tempted to forge ahead and let normal training resume. I wasn't injured, so in my mind there was nothing to stop me from running, but I had to listen to the data. My heart rate variability was still raised and my inflammation levels were extremely elevated. Pushing through would put greater stress on my body, delaying my recovery – it would take eight weeks for them to return to normal.

As someone who finds it hard to sit still (having got to this point in in my story you're probably not surprised by that), I filled my recovery with social activities and work instead. I spent time catching up with friends, drinking a little too much wine, pushing ahead on SheRACES projects (lots of meetings with global sports organisations and race directors) and giving my body a rest. I had taken on two huge challenges within the space of nine months and I just needed normal life to resume. My head longed for a break from spreadsheets, splits and logistics planning, and I just wanted to enjoy a long, slow run on the trails fuelled by Twix bars and flapjacks.

But I was caught in a dichotomy. I needed to run to clear my head, de-stress and problem-solve, but I found it difficult to be motivated without a race or challenge on the horizon. I couldn't just sign up for anything, though. It had to have purpose behind it; a strong 'why' to enable me to fully commit. Everyone kept asking what I was going to do next. It was like the pressure parents feel to have a second child: as soon as you've had your first — everyone expects you to do it all over again and I was expected to do something bigger, badder, tougher, longer, faster. But I wasn't chasing Instagram likes or Strava kudos — I was pursuing something more important than my personal goals.

And so it became a time to pause for thought, take stock of what running meant to me and what I had learned so far. There was a limit to the number of matches I could burn in my life. Cambodia had been the first, followed by Ireland, and then the treadmill. It was not sustainable to do harder and harder challenges to fundraise for SheRACES to support our work and to try to inspire others, because, ultimately, where would that stop? And at what cost to my body? Like Edda Bauer, who I met in Cambodia and Bhutan, I wanted running to be part of my life for as long as possible, but running was also now intrinsically linked with my desire to drive change.

Fifteen years ago, on the sandy start line of Marathon des Sables, I was on an entirely different journey. I was curious about taking on tough challenges, signing up for race experiences that sung to me or catapulted me into far-flung places I wanted to explore. It was a highly personal pursuit. I was running to escape the rat race and chase the endorphin rush, but there was no big-picture thinking.

Looking back at the photo of me feeding Cormac at UTMB, I began to wonder what would have happened if I had stayed silent; if I had simply returned to my life as a tech CEO and hadn't followed my gut instinct to take the opportunity to create a platform. What if I hadn't been strong enough to give up my high-flying career and do what I loved most, which was to help others? Where would I be? I certainly wouldn't be a GB runner, and probably not a mother of three. It was stepping back from corporate life and becoming my own boss which gave me the confidence that our lives had room for Saoirse, our third child, without taking away from the boys. It enabled me to have more flexibility to train and take on challenges with a purpose. It allowed me to create SheRACES and advocate for others.

From that moment in the Alps when Alexis approached me, camera in hand, my life changed. I had shared my story, my struggles with pregnancy and prolapse, and begun the first baby steps towards empowering women to lead active lives. As I took time to recover and reflect on my life through the lens of running, I felt tremendously grateful for the education and upbringing which gave me the confidence to use my voice. I may have faced barriers, but I was still in a very privileged position. Many women face far greater barriers than me, and I was incredibly lucky to have access to the countryside from an early age and the means to change my career. I will never have first-hand experience of being a woman of colour, a survivor of domestic violence or someone living with neurodiversity or a limiting medical condition; but via SheRACES I can open up conversations to include these women with lived experience, actively pulling up a seat to the table when they don't have one. It may have started with pregnancy deferrals and my own story, but it soon became about so much more.

Within three years SheRACES has gone from talking about normalising the stocking of period products at race aid stations to driving change across the globe. We're having an impact on, and working with, sporting bodies and global race companies in India, Uzbekistan, Oman, Turkey, USA, Hong Kong and more. UTMB, Ironman, England Athletics, Athletics Ireland, British Triathlon and the Pro Trail Runners Association have all sought our advice to improve the experience for female athletes. Some race directors have been motivated to improve conditions for women because it is simply the right thing to do. But for others I've had to prove that doing the right thing also increases the bottom line.

Things were starting to change. SheRACES was empowering women to speak up, be assertive and challenge the normal way of doing things. I was no longer having to call out races on their behalf – women were doing it for themselves, with increasing numbers of men as our allies. Race policies had changed; marketing campaigns had shifted to a female focus and elite athletes were starting to speak out. And the repercussions were far wider than running. I started to use the lens of sport as a way to change patriarchal attitudes towards women. I was invited to work on a maternity policy with Brentford Football Club, not for their athletes, but for their season ticket holders. It was no longer just about getting women on start lines and creating equality in sport; it was about access to medical care, the right research into female bodies, support from the workplace, support from partners, sharing caring responsibilities and enabling women to become decision-makers. It was about understanding how inclusion equals profit and the framework which can facilitate this. Using the resilience and doggedness I gained from running, while leveraging the business skills I developed in my corporate career, I have been able to forge a new path through life.

It hasn't been an easy ride. I naively thought that presenting a case that women deserve to be equitably treated would be very simple. It's not just the right thing to do – it's good for business, as shown by our work with Threshold Sports (just a 1.5% increase in cost for their 50:50 ultra project had almost 100% more women on the start line, as well as an increase in men from the resulting publicity).

We still face pushback from those who want to maintain the status quo and continue being the gatekeepers of sport; those who have never faced barriers themselves and who won't accept that barriers exist for others. These are often younger women, women I recognise my younger self in. Before I was made redundant and told to have babies, I too believed that being a woman was not a barrier to success and can imagine myself questioning those using it as 'an excuse'. But there are also those who have been able to climb the barriers and are not willing to lower the ladder to other women. They have fought through and want other women to have to do the same. Calling for simple changes – like smoothing cut-offs to allow for a consistent pace, or separate female swim starts or changing areas – is inconsistent with their idea that we compete equally against men. The idea that every single woman should have the opportunity to participate is against their belief that only the strongest should survive. For me this has been diffi-cult to stomach at times. I've been told many times I'm a 'deep empath', which makes sense, as I struggle to understand how people cannot care for the experiences of others, and I feel so strongly driven to eliminate inequalities. It is also the reason I struggle to set boundaries and will prioritise helping an athlete with a problem over getting a proper night's sleep.

But these difficulties are much outweighed by the intense fulfilment I have experienced from helping others, as well as the incredible, deep relationships I have made with so many people - men and women - around the world who share my goals and support me in driving ever forwards. There is still so much to do and the finish line for SheRACES is only when it doesn't need to exist anymore – and I'll keep going until it does.

At the beginning of 2025, in the months following the treadmill record, I sat down to write this book. With no race or world record on the immediate horizon, I had time to reflect and think. I was physically strong and well recovered. My prolapse had settled and I knew I could run with confidence. Yes, there were more countries to run across, but there was no rush. It was time to consider what running really meant to me. As I began spooling over old diaries, blogs and race reports, I realised running had been the conduit for so much transformation in my life – from the anxious, overweight schoolgirl who was embarrassed to run in front of her peers to the strong woman who fought off sexist bullshit to conquer Spartathlon. The photograph of me breastfeeding mid-ultramarathon ultimately led to a life of advocacy, relinquishing my high-pressure career – for now at least – to pursue a more meaningful path. Running had created so much positive change in my life that I wanted to pay it forward, and SheRACES was the manifestation of this dream.

Reflecting back, I realise now that SheRACES wasn't born in a vacuum. I grew up watching my parents give their time freely to others – and it instilled a set of values in me. I always knew it was important to help others – to support women and be charitable – and it's a value that still drives me today. Now, as I move into my forties with two running world records under my belt, I have the credibility to talk about resilience, goal setting and driving positive change to schoolchildren, athletes and business leaders alike. I'm always looking to deliver positive change in the world of business, as well as in sport, and I've been invited into the inner circles of prominent conferences, podcasts and industry events. My work has become informed by my running, rather than running being an escape away from my desk. But ultimately there was no escaping the question: what next?

Fortunately, I didn't have to wait too long for an answer. In May 2025 I received confirmation that I had been selected to represent Great Britain at the 24 Hour World Championships in Albi, France – and this time GB were taking a full six-female squad. It would be my third GB vest, but the first time I truly felt I deserved to be there. Rather than a looming sense of imposter syndrome I was excited to perform and finally feel part of the team. I could now pay it forward to that insecure teenager who never thought she was a runner – but it goes beyond that. This would be my moment to say to Saoirse and all the young girls around the world: 'You are strong, you are powerful, you belong.'

I've been stacking my bricks for over a decade and it is time to give it my all, but what does this mean in practice? I'm not a professional or sponsored athlete. This became crystal clear when I sent my friend Camille Herron a message. She replied: 'I'll get back to you after my nap.' Rest is part of her working day as a pro athlete, but to me it is a luxury I simply can't afford. Camille's life centres on being the best athlete she can possibly be, while mine is a balance of family, work and advocacy, alongside my athletic goals. Training is about doing as much as I can within significant constraints. I simply can't compare myself to those whose job it is to run. Doing my absolute most is about 80 per cent on the Tom Evans spectrum. I can never train 100 per cent, but I can train smart and optimise my time. My life has so many dimensions to it and I can never know what a life dedicated to performance would be like.

It is an absolute lie that you can 'have it all.' It is impossible to be fully committed to more than one thing at a time. And anyway, I wouldn't be happy giving over that last 20 per cent to training, because I would always be happier channelling it into my family and giving others the opportunities that I have had. Giving 100 per cent would leave my life without purpose or balance. I just have to stop comparing myself to others, because the only comparison I can make is with myself. My goal is to give my best performance, but not worry about placements or rankings. I have to be honest about what I can achieve given the time and resources I have, but I have come to realise over time that I want an array of strings holding me up.

When I was young my career was the only thread. When this was violently cut I had nothing to keep me from falling – until I found Muay Thai and then running. In order to thrive, I need multiple threads. This means I can cope if one snaps, because I have many fulfilling strands to my life. I am not one thing. I am a business woman, an advocate, a mother, a wife and a runner. I have many places to draw confidence from and my identity no longer relies on just one aspect.

But with this multifaceted identity comes many complications. The question I am asked most is 'How do you juggle it all? The kids, the running, work, fighting for change – just where do you find the time?' Throw into the mix increased training for the World Championships and it's enough to make anyone question their life choices. The truth is, it's all about creative thinking. Depending on where I am in my training cycle, I tap into different lifelines. I'm fortunate to have a cleaner and the flexibility to work evenings and weekends, but even that wouldn't be enough without my village of friends who share childcare, swapping school runs so I can sneak in an extra-long session.

So here's how I do it. And if you have other tips and tricks I'm all ears – we're in this together and I'll share them to the world. For us, it all starts with a Sunday evening meeting between John and me over dinner. We track the whole family's movements across the next week: who needs to be where and when, and what (kids') sporting and social fixtures are on, before working out where training slots can fit. John's out of the door for work by 6 a.m. in the week, so dawn runs aren't an option, unless I'm on our turbo trainer or treadmill at home. I often prefer to work out in the evenings, though. It's not uncommon for me to be found on the treadmill or bike at 9 p.m. replying to work emails, or in the infrared sauna, cranking out heat training miles on the bike to boost my red blood cell count. Most weeks I can commit to training six days, with Friday sacred for Mummy and Saoirse time (she is at nursery at least half days the rest of the week while her brothers are at school). I'm walking 15 miles a week up and down hills just ferrying the kids to school – miles that count toward my training. I usually run straight from school drop-off in the mornings before I start work, and if we have a family outing planned at the weekend I'll lace up and run to meet them, sending a change of clothes, recovery fuel and a big flask of tea in the car. As chief family organiser I definitely choose the location to fit the distance I want to run!

During school holidays I'll drop the kids at activity camps, leaving the car with them. I'll then run home before returning later, on foot, to collect the kids and car. At hockey or tennis matches you'll see me doing circuits around the pitch or courts; when they're biking I'll run intervals, trying to keep up, pausing only to dole out snacks. My coach Eddie – also a mum of three and juggling wizard – builds my recovery weeks around school holidays and fine-tunes workouts to fit this unpredictable, glorious chaos. I save even more time by living almost entirely in Lycra, rarely wearing make-up or 'doing' my hair, batch-cooking meals and banana flapjacks, and teaching the kids to tackle tasks themselves. It not only builds great resilience, but means I spend less time chasing around after them. When my eldest was too lazy to pack his own swimming bag for school I put in a bright pink Disney princess towel we'd been handed down. He's never asked me to pack his bag since.

When I'm in my normal base training phase, I hover around 100km a week – enough to keep the wheels turning without tipping me over the edge. But for the World Championships I have to dial everything up: more kilometres, heavier strength sessions, smarter recovery. Now 10 weeks out as I write this, I'll slowly ramp from that comfy 100km to peak at a hefty 150km per week. It's a bonkers routine – one I couldn't sustain year-round – but it's a commitment the whole family rallies behind for a season. To fit in that hefty mileage count I'll throw in some training races along the way. It means I can carry less gear and have water and aid stations at my disposal. A few weeks back I ran 100km in the Threshold Race to the Stones event. It was a boiling hot day, temperatures reaching 33 degrees and I knew I had to rely on data to manage my performance. I still don't have time to train as much as others, so taking a scientific approach to heat adaption, cooling and fuelling, helps me to optimise every part of my training. On this particular day, I was not racing to win, I just needed to have a strong training run and not overcook myself. The aim was to have the fastest training run I could, but still be able to run again two days later. To keep myself in check, I had a CORE temperature sensor fitted to my arm which connected to my watch. I knew from running in the heat over the summer that if my temperature rose above 38.7 degrees I started to feel terrible and struggled to take on fuel. My goal was to keep my temperature below that marker, ideally around 38.5. I didn't look at my pace at all and had no idea where I was in the race. If my temperature rose above 38.7 I eased off, and if it dropped below 38.5 I pushed a little more. The metrics worked. I coped well in the heat and was surprised – and delighted – to turn the final corner and see tape across the finish line. I had come first, beating over 300 women and placing ninth overall out of over 1,000 runners! It was not my goal but it was a delicious cherry on top of a successful run (and I had a big trophy to take home to the kids). It demonstrated to me how far my performance has come and why in my forties I'm in the best shape of my life, ahead of hopefully my best World Champs.

Right now, I'm standing on the starting line of that build-up and the kids are buzzing with excitement. They've never seen me toe the line in a real, live World Championships, so having John and the three of them cheering me on in France is going to feel like the ultimate home-crowd advantage. But it's also a huge team effort and the kids are very much on board. Our garden turns into a plyometric playground, the kids racing me in burpee broad jumps (spoiler: they always win) and doubling as dumbbells during my strength sets, shrieking with glee every time I grunt. As training cranks up, I constantly juggle priorities, running a quick cost-benefit check on every minute. This means hitting the treadmill when the kids are asleep, pulling in more favours from mum friends, TV-binge workouts on the bike and planning family holidays to training-friendly destinations. My little family crew know that if their organisation slips, so does my iron-clad routine. It's a messy, manic compromise, but it works for us. Sure, workouts get missed and runs cut short, but I've learned that an 80 per cent effort on a day filled with laughter and chaos beats perfection every time. My secret weapon? Pure happiness. Sharing these sweaty, silly moments with my family fuels me more than any solo session ever could.

In the end, though, it's all noise – there's nothing left to prove. I'm not sure there ever has been, but I haven't known that until now. My performance is secondary to the story I'd tell my teenage self, the girl who never thought she was capable. Be proud of who you are. Do the uncomfortable. Test your limits. You can achieve so much more than you ever know and what matters is what your body can do, not what it looks like. I already see the ripples permeating through my own children. They identify as athletes, have confidence in their abilities and revel in the size of their growing muscles. They're the ones who care most about the World Championships, because finally they'll each have a GB vest to wear, as well as see their mummy race. I challenge myself in order to inspire them to become bold, strong and resilient individuals. But most of all I hope I have paved a way for my daughter to harness her own power. My biggest wish is that she enters a world where all girls and the women they become believe they belong in sport. In the end my legacy is to pay it all forward to Saoirse and her generation.

As for my personal goals, it's about one purposeful step at a time, choosing joy over pressure, savouring every sunset-soaked run instead of chasing accolades. There are still world records to be broken (of course I have a few adventures in mind – the kids want more for show-and-tell) but they are more about the experience than the result. As I nudge closer to perimenopause, I have no idea how my body will change, but I know I'll nurture it, keep lacing up, hoping to still be running decades from now. My future's a wide-open trail and I'm excited to see where it leads.

EPILOGUE

It's 2 August 2025. I've been standing on the finish line for over ten hours and will be here for another three – or whatever it takes. I'm not leaving until every woman has achieved her goal.

I wrote much of this book six years ago. At that point it ended with UTMB, when I began to tell my story in the hope of empowering other mothers across the world to set their own goals (as well as have more confidence to breastfeed in public). A moment like that doesn't come around more than once a lifetime. The race and that photo had surely created the most impact I could ever hope for, and I felt that this was my whole story and it was time to tell it.

But something felt wrong and I pressed pause. Somewhere inside I still believed I had another chapter to write; I just didn't know what it was. The story up until then hasn't changed, but I now very much feel it was the prologue. The photo wasn't the end, it was just a door opening into a new world, with new dreams to follow and fresh stories to write. I certainly didn't expect these stories to include running for my country, breaking world records or impacting millions of women – and yet they did.

When Charlotte (the lovely editor of this very book) approached me, mid-treadmill world record, asking me if I'd consider writing a book, the time finally felt right. Or perhaps I was too tired to say no! It felt right not because I don't have another chapter to write in the future – after all, who knows where life will take me from here – but it felt right because I wanted to do all I could to help others write another chapter in their lives.

As I stand here at the inaugural SheRACES 25k and 50k trail event finish line, women continue to stream over it. Some hand in hand with their children, some hand in hand with women they hadn't met until they started this race. They have bonded over their struggles, sharing life stories as they have made their way through 50km of undulating Peak District trails. Dads sit in the sun feeding babies or kicking footballs around with their toddlers. They have been patiently waiting for their partners to arrive. As I put the women's medals around their necks I ask about their journeys. Many have never entered an event before or run further than 5km. Now they have completed an ultramarathon and the feelings of elation are radiating from them for all to see. A woman with a crutch hiked the entire way while a young woman 22-weeks pregnant turned to this race because she had been rejected by others.

'I only started running in January and now I can call myself an ultrarunner,' a woman in her fifties told me.

'I've bloody done it – what an amazing experience,' said another woman in her late 60s.

The feeling of love and support is unlike any other race I've experienced. The mood is relaxed, and women hang around for hours to share their experiences with one another, rather than racing off home.

'I was always picked last in school sports,' one woman confides in another.

'Me too. But this was just what I needed,' her new friend replies.

I put my sunglasses on to hide my tears. I know what this achievement could mean for them, giving strength across their entire lives, just as my own running has done for me. All it took was putting on the right event, removing all the barriers we could and giving them the confidence to sign up. For many, their journey to this finish line has represented a new beginning in their lives, rewriting the limits that have held them back in the past, opening up new possibilities.

Two months later I'm standing in my white spaceman-like podium tracksuit, gold medal around my neck singing God Save the King. Actually, I'm singing God save the Queen as my sleep deprived state has made me forget we've moved on another Royal generation. Two hours previously our GB women's team became 24 Hour World Champions, setting a new team World Record, and my incredible teammate Sarah Webster recording a new individual world record of 278.622 kilometres (173.127 miles) at the age of 46.

My kids are at the side of the ceremony watching on. School had given a rare 'authorised absence' for a day off for them to watch me represent our country and I can see in their faces what this moment means to them.

For me it wasn't the perfect race. But in some ways it was the race I truly wanted. The race where I would have to dig in deeper than ever to achieve a shared goal.

———

Standing on the start line, ice bandana around my neck to precool my body, I take in a deep breath. I have to focus. I call my five teammates into a huddle. We're all running in the individual race, but we're also running as a team, where our top three distances over the 24 hours are added together for team medals. We speak about how we're ready. How we will go out and fight for one another on course. I feel part of a team, a sisterhood, in the way that I never have before in running.

Sixteen hours in and I'm tracking exactly on target. As usual I've broken up the 24 hours into 8 x 3-hour blocks, all with a target pace that gets slower each block (240km target which starts at 8.30-minute miles, ending at 10.30s, assuming 30 minutes of pee and admin stops). We're running a 1.5km loop around a park in Albi, France, partly on a track but then on concrete paths round football pitches and sports buildings. I'm fuelling well

– mostly on jam sandwiches (made into little bread parcels with my toastie device), jelly babies and gels.

It's 2 a.m. and I'm feeling the sleepiness kick in. For a second, I lose concentration and take a bad line, stumbling over some uneven concrete. My right hip flexor starts to seize up, making running painful and laboured. Damn it. It was all going so well. In any other race I would just have stopped. There would be no point making an injury worse for another eight hours. But I'm third counter for the team after Kelsey Price and Sarah, and we're currently in gold medal position. Quitting is not possible.

I have to recalculate. If we're going to have a chance of winning the team medal I can't risk falling again so I take a five-minute powernap (followed by another one later), then a quick physio treatment. In my head, each time I stop I'm wasting precious personal kilometres, but I have to remind myself my personal target is secondary to the team goal. Ali Young and Joasia Zakrzewski are in fourth and fifth placing on our team but still running well. They take turns to pace me, letting me settle behind them, wincing as I do. I just have to maintain this pace and with Kelsey and Sarah running so well, Gold is surely ours. At 8.a.m, with two hours to go, my kids arrive back to the track, Cormac shouting his 'you're flying round the track like a rockstar' chant. I try to hold back my tears and smile as I pass them each lap, letting go of my emotions when I turn the corner. I don't know how far we are ahead of the Aussies, who are in second place – we can only see individual scores each lap – so I have to keep pushing for the team, but it's a pain I've never felt before.

I get told with only minutes to go that we've definitely secured the Gold. We're actually 20-odd kilometres in total ahead of the Aussies and it's a World Record team performance. Ali and I walk the last home straight so we finish in front of my family who are cheering from the stands. The last thing you want to do in a 24-hour race is finish at the furthest point on the lap from your crew when the gun goes and then have to waddle back! It's a weird feeling not achieving my personal goals – I'm 3km short of my PB, and 7km short of my target – but I'm still on top of the world. For once in my career this hasn't been about me and my goals but running for others, which helped me push harder than I ever have before. As we embrace as a team, I feel a huge sense of gratitude for these incredible women helping unlock another level inside me.

As I look down at that medal on stage, I think about this book, and how I've ended this extra chapter I never believed I'd have. The journey from hobby-runner to World Champion. I'd never have believed it when that UTMB photo was taken.

After the ceremony, our team poses for photos while my four-year-old runs laps of the track because she wants to be like her mummy. The boys are arguing over who gets the medal first for show and tell. Four of the six of us are mums and we share stories of how our children think differently to their peers as to what is possible for them. I'm nauseous. I haven't eaten in the four hours since the race ended and I'm trying to get a single salt and vinegar Pringle into my mouth just to start refuelling. It's 2 p.m. on Sunday, and I've had two five-minute naps since Saturday morning. But despite this, my mind is racing. If this is the end of this chapter, then what comes after?

I think of the women at the SheRACES Trail Series, achieving their goals and expanding their horizons for the future. I don't know what lies next for me. But I know I have more barriers to break down, more stories to tell and more trails to conquer.

We all have another chapter to write. Our lives until now have just been preparing us for it. Crossing a finish line isn't always the end. It can be just the beginning.

ACKNOWLEDGEMENTS

Writing this book has been an ultramarathon in itself, one that would not have been possible without the support, encouragement and inspiration of many incredible people. I am possibly the last person my English teacher ever expected to write a book – me being the only one in our year 10 class who dared argue that we should have more IT classes and less English literature. I guess I'm also almost the last person my PE teacher expected to represent our country at running so perhaps I'm just a natural outlier.

Charlotte and all the team at Bloomsbury – thank you for approaching me in my moment (48 hours) of weakness on the treadmill, and convincing me that writing a book is easier than running an ultramarathon. It is now clear that it is definitely far harder, but I'm so grateful for the support you have given in helping me get my story out to the world and hopefully inspiring others to write new chapters in their lives.

Lily – without you this book may never have seen the light of day (or at least taken a few more years). Thank you for all the incredible hard work in helping me shape my story and get this across the finish line. We have to be friends forever as you know too much about me!!! Thank you also to Louise and Stephanie for reading this and your insightful feedback.

Alexis – this is all your 'fault'! Without your incredible photographic eye I would probably still be working long hours as a CEO or CFO, never having represented my country at running and a mother of 2, not 3. To have you photograph Saoirse crossing the line at TDS with me was incredibly special and I am forever indebted to you for the life I now lead.

To 'Team Sophie' – Brendan, Lucy, Brett for getting me ready for every start line (and patched up after every finish). Eddie – you are the most incredible coach and friend – I am so inspired by you and grateful for the trail you have laid for me to achieve more than I ever believed. To my incredible village around me, especially Claire and Ciara for taking my kids in with yours when I need time to train (or to write!). I could not do what I do without you.

Mum and Dad – thank you for giving me every chance to grow and succeed, but always with the wisdom not to hand everything to me easily. I would not have achieved what I have if you did. Watching you embrace your roles as grandparents has brought me so much joy, and I am thankful for the support you continue to give our family.

To my wonderful children, Donnacha, Cormac and Saoirse – you are my daily inspiration, reminding me that there are no limits except those we set ourselves. Your boundless energy, curiosity, kindness and joy fill my life and keep me on my toes. I am so excited to see where life takes you.

To my beloved John – saying yes to a lifetime together remains the best decision I have ever made. Every day, I am amazed by your love, strength, and commitment to our family. Your belief in me has helped me dream beyond limits and reach goals I never imagined. I am endlessly grateful for you and the life we share together.

To the SheRACES community and all the women who have shared their stories: Your courage and honesty have inspired me to use my voice for change. Thank you for trusting me with your experiences and for joining me in the fight for equality in sport. To Julie, Anna, Sophie and all those who have given their time and funds to support SheRACES I am truly grateful. We have so much work to do but we have the momentum to achieve it.

To the race organisers and advocates who are working for a better future: Thank you for listening, learning, and striving to make sport more inclusive. Your willingness to challenge the status quo gives me hope for the next generation of athletes. (Oh, and for those who have stood in my way; you may have thought you were creating barriers, but I have grown stronger from having to climb them so I guess I should thank you as well).

To my running friends – I never imagined that signing up to my first ultra would have led to lifelong friendships across the world. I value these far more than any medal, trophy or accolade.

And finally, to every runner, parent, and advocate who dreams of a more equitable sporting world. This book is for you. May we continue to run towards change - together.

With gratitude,
Sophie x
www.sheraces.com

RACES

To the best of my knowledge, this list covers every marathon and ultra I've run. But since not all my races make it onto Strava, I can't swear it's exhaustive – think of it as 'mostly comprehensive with a small chance of accidental omissions'.

2009
Run to the Beat Half Marathon 21.1km
XNRG Druid's Challenge 136km

2010
Northampton to Tring 45 miles
Tring to Northampton 45 miles
XNRG Pilgrim Challenge 53km (DNF)
Marathon des Sables 250km

2011
Northampton to Tring 45 miles
Racing the Planet Nepal 220km
Ironman Switzerland

2012
Go Beyond Country to Capital 43 miles
Northampton to Tring 45 miles
Go Beyond Thames Trot Ultramarathon 47 miles
Centurion Thames Path 100 miles
Comrades Marathon 87km
Challenge Vichy 70.3 Triathlon
Fire + Ice Iceland 250km
Global Limits Cambodia 220km (DNF)

2013
Go Beyond Country to Capital 43 miles
Go Beyond Thames Trot Ultramarathon 47 miles
Global Limits Bhutan 200km

2014
Go Beyond Country to Capital 43 miles
XNRG Pilgrim Challenge 53km

2015
Centurion North Downs Way 50 miles
Chiltern 50 Ultra Challenge 50km
Round the Rock Ultramarathon 48 miles
Ultra Tour Monte Rosa 170km
Grand 2 Grand Ultra 270km
Centurion Autumn 100 miles

2016
Go Beyond Country to Capital 43 miles
Transgrancanaria 130km
Centurion North Downs Way 50 miles
Centurion South Downs Way 50 miles
Centurion South Downs Way 100 miles
Marathon du Medoc 42.2km
Spartathlon 246km

2017
Go Beyond Country to Capital 43 miles
Phoenix Marathon
Testway Ultra 46.5 miles
Gran Trail Courmayeur 105km (DNF – 75km course completed)

2018
Ultra Trail du Mont Blanc 171km

2019
Go Beyond Country to Capital 43 miles
Impact Marathon Guatemala 42.2km
North Downs Way 50 miles
Summer Spine Race 268 miles

Phoenix Trail Marathon
Battersea 24 Hour Track
Mince Pie Run 31 miles

2020
Go Beyond Country to Capital 43 miles

2021
North Downs Ridge 50km
XNRG Pilgrim Challenge 53km
London Marathon 42.2km
Lakeland 100 miles
Maverick South Downs 50km

2022
Punchbowl Marathon
The Fox 62km
Phoenix 24 Hour Track
South Downs Way 100
Verona 24 Hour World Championships
Centurion Wendover Woods 50 miles
Impact Marathon Scotland

2023
6 Hour Phoenix Track Wars
Crawley 24 Hour Track
Eiger Ultra-Trail by UTMB
Taiwan 24 Hour World Championships

2024
Ireland World Record
TDS (Sur les Traces des Ducs de Savoie) by UTMB 148km
SheUltra 50km
Centurion Wendover Woods 50 miles (DNF)

2025
Treadmill 48 Hour World Record
Phoenix Trail Marathon
Race to the Stones 100km
Pilgrims Trail Marathon
Albi 24 Hour World Championships